CW01551432

just one thing

VOLUME TWO

just one thing

VOLUME TWO

40 Daily Habits for Better Health

contents

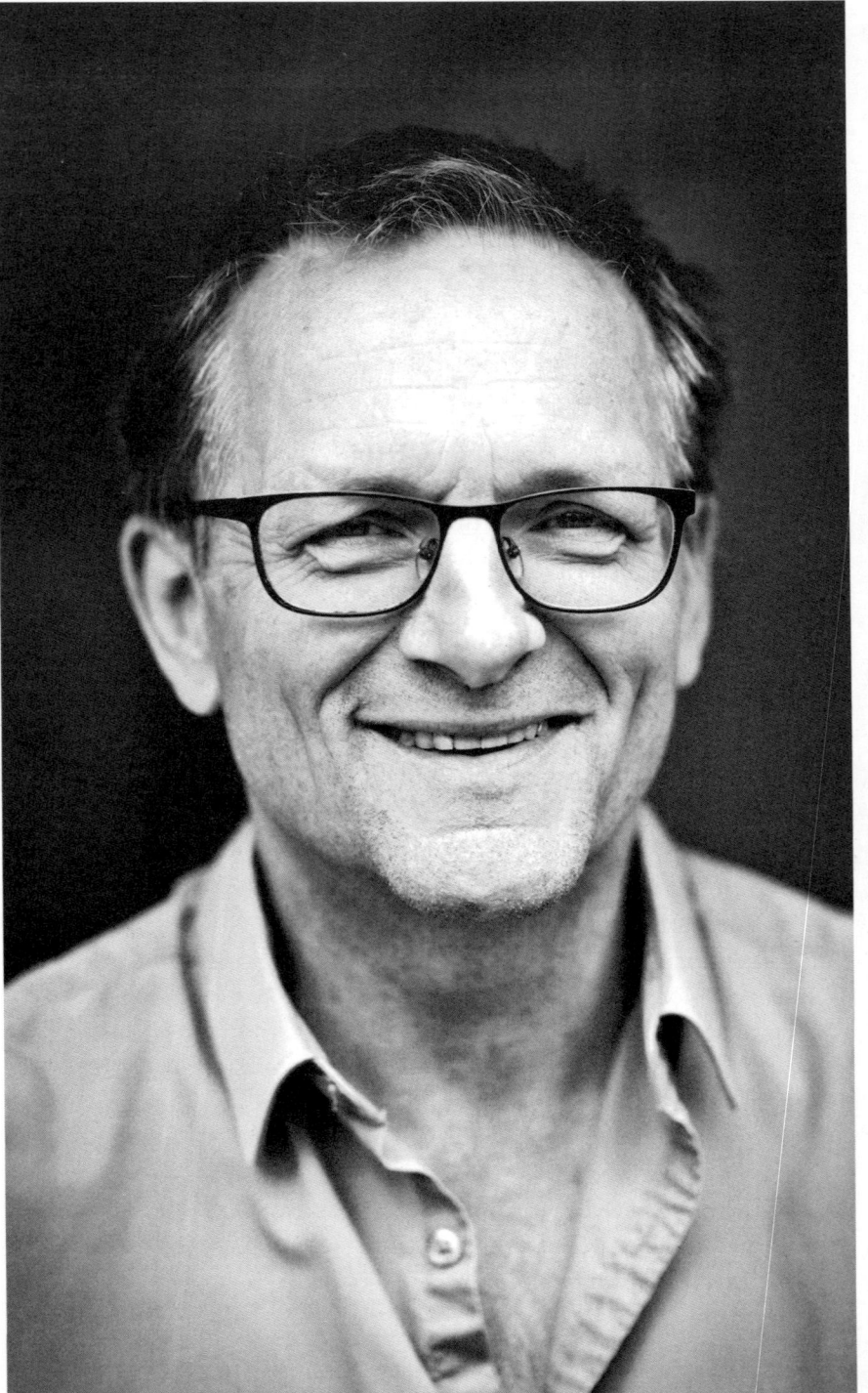

Foreword

BY CLARE BAILEY MOSLEY AND JACK MOSLEY

CLARE: The outpouring of grief when Michael died of heatstroke on a hillside in Greece in June 2024, one of the hottest recorded days, was extraordinary. The family and I were deeply touched by the warmth and kindness of the *Just One Thing* community. So many people shared how they had benefitted from Michael's advice, and how he was like a friend to them.

Michael personally understood the challenges of pursuing a healthy and happy lifestyle, having struggled himself with his weight, diabetes and chocolate addiction. He would ask me to hide the chocolate to avoid temptation. Only a few months ago, a large bar of hidden chocolate fell off the shelf with a heavy clunk onto my desk! Yet, through his curiosity, research and clarity, along with an excellent team around him, he was able to help make healthy change achievable – JUST ONE THING at a time!

Michael was always passionate about supporting the nation's health, knowing that so many of the chronic conditions that cause poor metabolic health across the Western world can be addressed by simple lifestyle changes. Our son Jack and I share this passion, and Jack has helped me pick up Michael's work where he left off. Jack is a GP registrar with an interest in diabetes, weight loss and chronic disease, and has recently published a bestselling book, *Food Noise*. How proud Michael would have been.

Ever since 2012, when Michael brought his type 2 diabetes into remission using intermittent fasting, he took it upon himself to inspire people worldwide to make lifestyle changes to improve their health. However, he understood that we are often overloaded with lifestyle advice that can become overwhelming: how to sleep better, how to control your anxiety, what foods to eat, what foods not to eat, how to lose weight, the best way to exercise.

Michael believed that willpower was overrated. However, he understood the power of habit and the benefit of breaking down those lifestyle tips into bitesized chunks. That was one of the reasons why *Just One Thing* was so well loved, not just in the UK, but around the world. Through *Just One Thing*, Michael may well have improved the health of hundreds of thousands, if not millions, of lives across the globe.

I am so delighted that *Just One Thing Volume 2* has been published, albeit posthumously.

JACK: The simplicity of *Just One Thing*, as well as my dad's infectious enthusiasm and passion, meant that it was a phenomenal hit. He had a fantastic ability to break down complex scientific research and to communicate in such an understandable and interesting way.

Having such an amazing archive of material, from *Just One Thing* to his many TV programmes, felt like a blessing to our family in the aftermath of Dad's passing. After he died, it took months before I felt able to watch or listen to anything he had produced. Eight months after he died, I started to relisten to his *Just One Thing* podcast and I was immediately hooked. Although it was emotionally difficult to listen at first, I was struck by the wealth of useful, evidence-based and easy-to-action information. It is a treasure trove of tips for people wanting to make small changes to their lives. The beauty of *Just One Thing* is that those changes, though seemingly small, have an incredible cumulative effect on helping you live a happier, healthier and more productive life!

My dad's authenticity was a great part of his appeal, and a reason why *Just One Thing* meant so much to him and why it was such a great fit. For much of his life, he was far from perfect when it came to looking after his health. He had a sweet tooth and was likely addicted to chocolate. He struggled with insomnia, and would be the first to admit he was no lover of exercise. This meant that he really did understand what others were going through and meant he truly could empathise. I suspect it made him more passionate about improving the nation's health, and figuring out ways to incorporate these changes so that they were not too much of a chore, and became a habit.

Over the last decade, there has been a staggering growth in interest in the 'wellness industry' worldwide. Through *Just One*

Thing, Michael was on hand to cut through the noise, and help provide guidance on what really works and what is just hot air. Through the podcast, he met many renowned scientists who were performing cutting-edge research into an area of medicine that had been previously left by the wayside: lifestyle medicine. He found it fascinating, and was always sharing a story or an interesting piece of research. The last conversation I had with him was a long chat on the phone, which finished with him enthusiastically telling me about the latest way to exercise: Nordic walking!

His love for the topics he discussed really shone through. He left a lasting impression on so many. Who isn't still brushing their teeth on one leg? He will be missed by many across the world, who felt like they had lost a friend when he died. Just One Thing we can take away from all this is the phenomenal legacy he leaves. It is not just the impact he had on his family and those who knew him, but on the many millions across the world. His legacy lives on and we are delighted to introduce this brilliant new book – *Just One Thing Volume 2* – so that you can continue to improve your life bit by bit through the learnings of *the one and only* Dr Michael Mosley. Here are 40 slices of simple, accessible and actionable advice you can slot into your life and, piece by piece, make real and lasting improvements. While these 'things' featured on dad's podcast, they have never before been published in book form. So what are you waiting for? Dive into this book and uncover what really works.

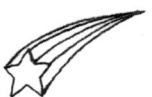

Introduction

Just One Thing has become a remarkable worldwide success. Originally launched as a BBC Radio 4 podcast in 2021, the series – a bitesized format offering single, manageable health tips, one at a time – has now reached more than 25 million listeners worldwide.

The idea is wonderfully simple: each 15-minute episode introduces Just One Thing you can do to improve your health. The series is full of quirky, fun and sometimes bizarre facts, and words of fascinating wisdom from eminent, and often very entertaining, scientists who are experts in their field.

In each episode, the researchers find a brave volunteer to give the 'thing' a test run. Of course, many people will associate the clever *Just One Thing* format with the instantly recognisable voice of medical journalist Dr Michael Mosley, who started presenting the first *Just One Thing* podcasts from a makeshift studio in his bedroom wardrobe during lockdown.

Indeed, Michael was the front man for seven series of the podcast, enthusiastically extolling the virtues of standing on one leg, taking an afternoon nap or walking in the rain, and, true to character, he always tried each 'thing' himself. Filming for a TV series of *Just One Thing* was already underway when his life was very sadly cut short in the summer of 2024 at the age of 67.

Michael was passionate about distilling scientific information and showing people how to improve their health, and even though he is no longer around to present future podcasts, *Just One Thing* will continue, and his legacy lives on in so many ways.

The first *Just One Thing* book was published in 2023 and was based on the tips from the first 30 podcast episodes. It's changed countless lives in far-flung corners of the world, after topping the bestseller charts and being translated into 11 languages. Now the same team is proud to be bringing you Volume 2: an in-depth and up-to-date compilation of the amazingly beneficial science behind simple, easy lifestyle changes which appeared in the subsequent 40 podcast episodes.

In these pages, you'll learn some surprisingly simple hacks that you can easily fit into your day. Did you know that eating reheated pasta or rice (see page 157) can reduce levels of systemic inflammation (a body-wide immune response, often initially triggered by infection, injury or irritation) and lower your risk of heart disease, autoimmune disorders, obesity and bowel cancer? Or that sipping green tea (see page 75) can improve your mood as well as your heart health and helps to protect the brain from cognitive decline? Perhaps you've heard that breathing through your nose rather than your mouth (see page 89) is good for you, but did you realise that it increases oxygen uptake and can improve your gum health as well as your immunity and memory? There's something for everyone in the pages that follow, no matter your age or your fitness level.

A big part of the appeal of *Just One Thing* is its simplicity, and the way each 'thing' offers an intriguing way to turn good intentions into sustainable habits. The charm and relatability of this format is the way it manages to distil behavioural science into achievable actions, exemplifying how small changes can make a significant difference.

After all, most of us recognise the importance of keeping to a healthy weight, eating well, doing regular exercise, reducing stress and getting a good night's sleep. So what stops us? Well, first, we are bombarded on a daily basis by a lot of vague and often conflicting advice in newspapers, on social media and on TV: drink coffee, don't drink coffee, cut down on fat, eat more fat, get out in the sun, cover up with sunscreen, exercise slowly or step up the pace... Who to believe?

Then there is the problem of putting good advice into practice, of creating a new healthy habit and sticking to it. Many of us start off each new year resolved to be healthier and more active, but within a month or so most of us have returned to our previous way of life. This isn't because we are inherently lazy or weak-willed – it is because we haven't created the environment where a new habit will stick.

This book, like Volume 1, is all about quick and simple scientifically proven ways to improve health and wellbeing in a sustainable way. No one is expecting you to do all of them. Just pick and choose what works for you. The advantage of aiming for bitesized goals is that they will get you thinking, 'Okay, I could manage that,' and then, hopefully, you might find you are enjoying the activity and end up making it part of your life.

SOME RULES TO GET STARTED

If you genuinely want to make changes for the better and to improve your health, here are 10 rules, based on science, which you might find useful:

1. MAKE IT SIMPLE. The rationale behind *Just One Thing* is that you don't have to do a major overhaul of your life. The suggestions are things you can easily build into your routine. Small changes like switching off the noisy notifications on your phone, or breathing through your nose, really can yield big benefits in terms of better mood, improved sleep, a sharper brain and reduced disease risk.

2. BE REALISTIC. Begin by doing what you think you can manage; don't try to do all 40 'things' every day! Start small and build from there. You can always add in Just One More Thing later.

3. CREATE A TRIGGER. You're much more likely to stick with something if it is attached to an activity you are already doing: brushing your teeth, eating a meal or boiling the kettle, for instance. If you attach your new 'thing' to something you do every day, it is much more likely to stick as a habit.

4. KNOW WHY YOU ARE DOING IT. If you really understand the benefits of adopting a new habit, keep reminding yourself of these when you're tempted to give up. Knowing why something works will make you much more likely to stick to it. That's why this book contains lots of interviews with leading experts, as well as references to scientific studies, which are easy to look up online. Once you're convinced that these 'things' are worth doing and persisting with, you can tailor them to your own requirements.

5. STICK WITH IT FOR AT LEAST A MONTH. There is a widely held belief that you can introduce a new habit in 21 days. This is almost certainly untrue. A study published in the *European Journal of Social Psychology* concluded that it took anywhere between 18 and 254 days to ingrain a new habit.[1] Your stickability will depend on how easy and enjoyable you find the 'thing' and will be reinforced when you start to notice beneficial changes. So stick with it!

6. TRY TO SWAP BAD HABITS FOR GOOD ONES. Many bad habits are deeply ingrained and may feel almost impossible to shake, so it can be easier to try to swap them for better habits. This takes time and persistence, but it works! So, if you are in the habit of pouring yourself a beer (or two) when you relax in front of the TV in the evening, switch to red wine (one small glass only!) or swap the wine for a cup of decaffeinated tea.

7. TRY TO DO IT REGULARLY. Establishing a new habit is mainly about consistency and frequency. Although it is important to know why you are doing something, it is even more important to actually do it and do it on a regular basis. A lot of the things you will come across in this book can be done daily and sometimes even more than once a day. We have also tried to keep the things short, as the shorter something is, the more likely you are to stick to it. Just a few minutes a day is often all you need to see the benefits!

8. INVOLVE A FRIEND OR LOVED ONE. One of the main reasons why people pay for personal exercise trainers is that they feel they need someone around to make them stick to a plan. Doing a thing with a friend or loved one not only makes you more accountable, it can also make it more fun.

9. BE KIND TO YOURSELF. If you have found a thing that you really like the look of, but just can't stick to it, then perhaps it is not right for you right now. Don't beat yourself up: accept that this may not be the moment in your life when it works for you. Take a look through the book and see what else appeals to you. Or try something that might feel out of your comfort zone – you might surprise yourself!

10. KEEP A RECORD. Make a note of some of your health markers and measurements – such as your weight, your waist circumference, your heart rate, your blood pressure (equipment for this can be bought in a pharmacy or online) and your blood sugars (ditto). You may find it helpful to invest in a wearable tracker which monitors your steps and heart rate. Keeping a record and seeing your numbers change over time will show you how far you have come.

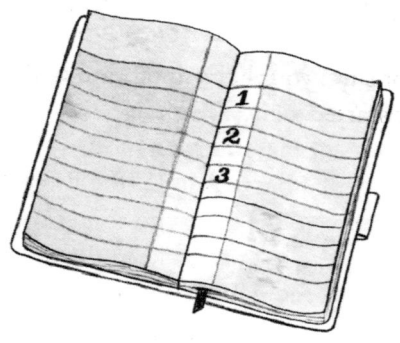

CHOOSING YOUR 'THING'

You'll find 40 fab 'things' to try in the following pages. Obviously, you don't need to try them all at once.

Many are so surprisingly brilliant that they have multiple potential benefits, boosting your heart health and your mood, or even extending your life, but we've arranged the chapters in this book under broad health headings. It's important to note that these chapter headings are simplified summaries and not medical claims.

So, if your primary concern is doing what you can to protect yourself from dementia, have a flick through the options in the Support Brain Health chapter across pages 48–93. Or if you are concerned about weight gain or type 2 diabetes, turn to the Manage Your Weight chapter from pages 130–67 first to see if there's any new habit you might be tempted to take on.

Start by trying one, then perhaps two, 'things' – and your confidence and commitment will grow. Once you've made your new 'thing' a habitual part of your life, browse the book again to see if there's another you fancy trying. Many can be easily done at intervals throughout your day, happily incorporated into your daily routine.

One thing is for sure: your body and brain will benefit hugely. So why not get started right away!

just one thing

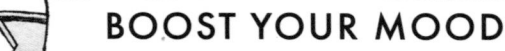

BOOST YOUR MOOD

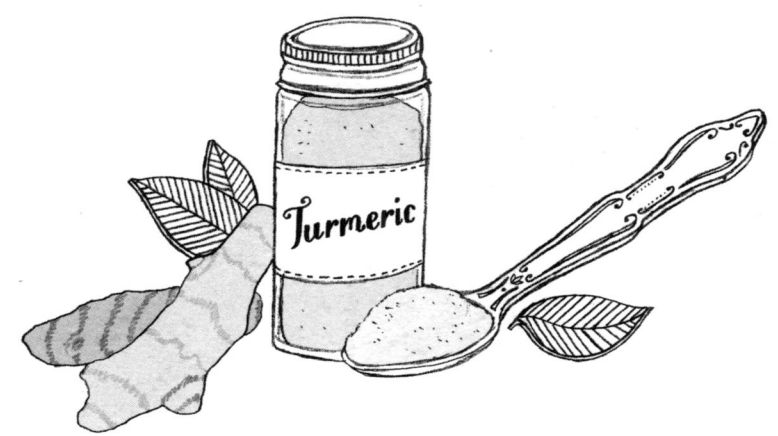

take turmeric

How to do it: Add one teaspoon of powdered turmeric to your cooking every day.

Why do it? It may boost mood, sharpen memory and help ease aches and pains.

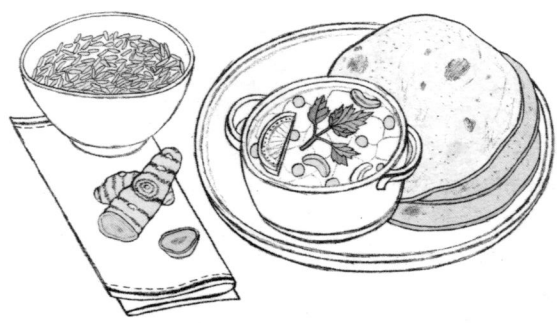

Next time you're cooking up a stew, soup or curry, consider adding a little something that could do more than just warm your taste buds.

Turmeric, with its distinctive golden hue, has long been a staple in kitchens across Southeast Asia. But increasingly, this pungent yellow spice is finding its way into the lexicons of scientists, doctors and wellness enthusiasts alike – not just for its flavour, but for its growing list of possible health benefits.

Most of us know turmeric as the dry, powdery spice that lends depth and colour to a curry. But if you come across it fresh, you'll find it's a relative of ginger, sharing that same gnarled appearance, with a pale brown skin that conceals a vivid, almost fluorescent yellow-orange interior. That striking colour comes from a compound called curcumin, the subject of hundreds of studies over recent decades, many of which suggest it may offer significant benefits for both body and brain.

Turmeric's use in medicine is nothing new. In fact, its therapeutic reputation stretches back thousands of years.

In Ayurvedic medicine, it was prescribed to ease liver complaints, digestive disorders, respiratory issues and even skin conditions. But modern science has recently started catching up, investigating whether there's truth to the age-old wisdom. And so far, the findings are compelling.

In 2022, a major Singaporean study[2] tracked nearly 2,700 older adults for five years. Those who regularly consumed turmeric – mainly in curry dishes – performed noticeably better on cognitive tasks than those who didn't. Their memory and problem-solving skills stayed sharper for longer. Researchers believe the secret lies in curcumin, a polyphenol (a type of plant-based compound) thought to reduce oxidative stress (a chemical imbalance that can lead to cell damage) and inflammation in the brain – both key contributors to cognitive decline.

Similar findings have emerged elsewhere. In Australia, a randomised trial[3] gave 80 adults a curcumin supplement and found measurable improvements in working memory and alertness. Volunteers also reported feeling less fatigued. It seems that turmeric may not only help with preserving cognitive ability but could also even give you a mental lift in the here and now.

TAMING INFLAMMATION

Much of turmeric's magic, scientists believe, lies in its ability to reduce inflammation. Inflammation is the immune system's response to infection, injury or irritation – and is a known factor in conditions ranging from heart disease to depression and cancer. In one Japanese study,[4] participants who took curcumin extract daily for several weeks showed significantly lower levels of C-reactive protein (CRP), a key marker of inflammation in the body. This anti-inflammatory effect has been particularly promising for people with joint pain and osteoarthritis, a condition affecting millions in the UK and around the world.

Dr Benny Antony, a senior research fellow at the Menzies Institute for Medical Research in Tasmania, has studied this area closely. 'Turmeric has been thought of as an anti-inflammatory agent for centuries,' he explains. 'It's also a powerful antioxidant and appears to have both antifungal and wound-healing properties.'

In one of his team's trials,[5] 70 participants with knee pain were split into two groups: one received a placebo, while the other took turmeric extract daily for 12 weeks. 'The results were encouraging,' says Dr Antony. 'Those taking turmeric experienced a greater reduction in pain and were able to cut back on their use of over-the-counter medications.'

Impressively, the turmeric group's improvements were comparable to those seen in patients taking ibuprofen. This is a potentially game-changing finding, especially for older adults or people with stomach issues who may not tolerate anti-inflammatory drugs well. Interestingly, scans and physical assessments showed that turmeric didn't appear to reduce inflammation directly inside the joint. This raises an important question: could it be working in a different way?

'There's a growing body of evidence suggesting turmeric may affect the gut–brain axis,' says Dr Antony. 'It appears to positively influence certain types of gut bacteria, which in turn may help regulate systemic inflammation. It's a more holistic kind of benefit – not necessarily targeting one site but working across the whole system.'

Of course, the Tasmanian trial was a small study, and turmeric should not be considered a substitute for prescribed medication. You should always seek medical advice before making changes to your treatment.

Though most studies have looked at people with chronic conditions like osteoarthritis, there's growing interest in turmeric's effect on acute pain, too. 'We believe it could have broader use, even in healthy individuals experiencing day-to-day aches and strains,' Dr Antony says. 'But more research is needed.'

OTHER BENEFITS

While brain and joint health are turmeric's headline acts, there are other emerging areas of interest. Curcumin has shown potential in managing metabolic syndrome, improving insulin sensitivity and helping regulate blood sugar levels. Some small-scale trials even suggest it may ease symptoms of asthma by dampening inflammation in the airways.

It's also under investigation for its potential role in preventing certain cancers, although findings are still preliminary. Lab studies[6] suggest curcumin can interfere with tumour cell growth and replication, but whether these effects carry over into real-world clinical outcomes remains uncertain. What we do know is that turmeric is generally safe. Side-effects are rare and typically mild – usually digestive, and only if taken in very large doses.

MAXIMUM ABSORPTION

One major challenge with turmeric is that it's not very well absorbed by the body on its own. That's why traditional cooking practices – often combining it with fat and other spices – may be more than just a happy accident.

'Curcumin is lipophilic,' says Dr Antony, 'meaning it dissolves in fat. You can boost absorption significantly by consuming turmeric with a little oil, and even more so if you add black pepper, which contains piperine. Piperine can increase curcumin absorption by up to 2,000 per cent.'

So cook it into a sauce or soup or stir it into full-fat yoghurt or milk to make a 'golden latte'. Just a teaspoon a day could make a difference.

FROM KITCHEN TO MEDICINE CABINET

Turmeric's transition from spice jar to health supplement is part of a broader shift towards more natural, food-based approaches to health. While it's unlikely to replace medicines or magic away chronic illness, it may offer a gentle, accumulative benefit over time.

For the everyday cook, the message is clear: don't be shy with turmeric. Whether you're stirring it into scrambled eggs, spooning it into your soup or sipping it in warm milk before bed, you're doing your body (and perhaps your brain) a favour.

There are few spices with such a rich combination of history, culinary versatility and promising health benefits. And with its golden glow and warming, earthy flavour, it's not a hard habit to acquire.

WHAT ABOUT A TURMERIC SUPPLEMENT?

Dr Antony believes turmeric supplements*, especially those containing piperine, are likely to deliver a more reliable dose if you're aiming for therapeutic effects. But not all supplements are created equal. Look for standardised extracts, preferably those combined with piperine, and always talk to your doctor if you're considering adding supplements to your daily routine – especially if you're on blood thinners or medication for diabetes.

* Just One Thing does not endorse any specific supplement or brand.

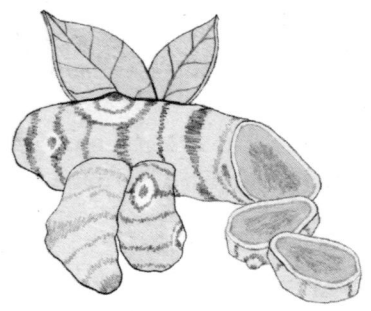

FIVE WAYS TO COOK WITH TURMERIC

Turmeric is one of the most versatile and forgiving ingredients in your spice rack. With its warm, earthy flavour and a hint of bitterness, it blends beautifully into a wide range of dishes – from hearty stews to delicate teas. Here's how to incorporate it effortlessly into your everyday cooking:

1. STIR INTO SOUPS AND STEWS. Add a teaspoon of ground turmeric to lentil soups, vegetable broths or slow-cooked curries. It provides depth of flavour and a vibrant colour. Sauté it briefly in oil first to release its aroma before adding liquids.

2. MAKE A GOLDEN LATTE. Also known as 'turmeric milk' or 'golden milk', this warming drink is perfect before bed. Whisk half a teaspoon of ground turmeric into warm milk (dairy or plant-based) with a pinch of black pepper, a grating of fresh ginger, a dash of cinnamon and a touch of honey.

3. ADD TO SCRAMBLED EGGS. For a breakfast boost, stir a small pinch of turmeric into your eggs as they cook. It won't overpower the flavour, but it will add a sunny colour and subtle complexity. A pinch of turmeric will add punch and vigour to an egg mayonnaise sandwich, too.

4. MIX INTO MARINADES AND RUBS. Combine turmeric with cumin, coriander, garlic, lemon juice and olive oil to make a simple rub for chicken, lamb or tofu. Allow the ingredients to marinate for at least an hour to absorb the flavour.

5. BRIGHTEN UP RICE OR COUSCOUS. Just a quarter teaspoon of turmeric in the cooking water will turn plain rice a brilliant yellow. Also add toasted nuts and herbs for a Middle Eastern twist.

TIP: Always cook turmeric with a little oil or fat and a pinch of black pepper to help your body absorb its active ingredient, curcumin, more effectively.

just one thing

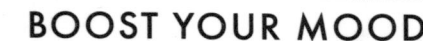

BOOST YOUR MOOD

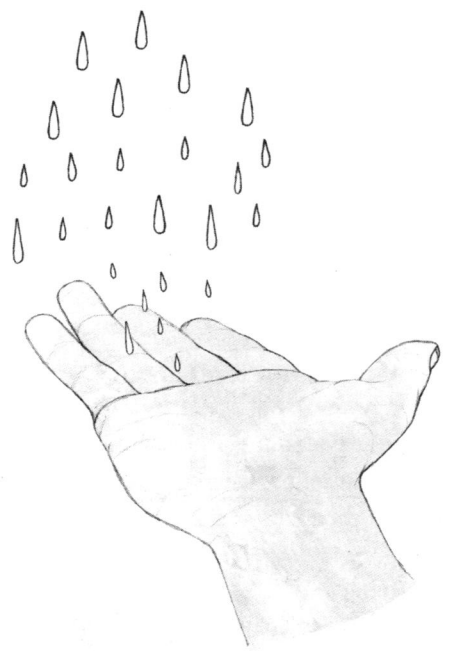

embrace the rain

How to do it: Go for a walk in the rain or head outside just after it's rained.

Why do it? It may reduce stress and inflammation while lifting your mood.

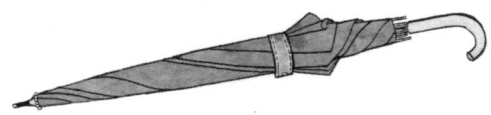

In the UK, it rains on 159 days of each year, on average. Rain is an unavoidable part of life – yet it is often unwelcome, frequently complained about and generally endured rather than enjoyed. But perhaps it's time that we changed our view of drizzle. Far from being a grey inconvenience, there's mounting scientific evidence that rain – and the air it leaves behind – may actually be good for us.

It's not just our gardens and farms that benefit from a good downpour. Rain helps to clean the atmosphere, flushing out pollutants and significantly improving air quality. One Japanese study[7] found that rainfall reduced the number of harmful fine particles in the air – the type that can lodge deep in the lungs – by around 20 per cent. This means that going for a walk in the rain, or shortly afterwards, doesn't just offer solitude and moody skies. It also delivers air that's cleaner and potentially better for your lungs than the air you'd breathe on a dry day in the city.

WHY RAINY AIR SMELLS SO GOOD
You may also have noticed the rich smell that follows rain falling on dry soil. That's called petrichor, a term coined in the 1960s, but understood for much longer by anyone who has stepped outside after a summer storm. The main chemical responsible is geosmin, a compound produced by soil-dwelling bacteria and released

into the air when raindrops hit dry ground. And it turns out that geosmin doesn't just smell good – it may make you feel good, too.

In a recent study from Korea,[8] researchers asked 30 healthy adults to handle soil containing geosmin, and compared various measures to those of a control group handling sterilised soil. After just five minutes of exposure, those in the geosmin group had elevated levels of serotonin – the mood-regulating neurotransmitter – in their blood. Brainwave activity also shifted into a more relaxed state, and their levels of C-reactive protein, a marker of inflammation (the immune system's response to injury, irritation or infection), fell. In other words, the smell of wet earth may have calming, anti-inflammatory effects on both brain and body.

While the air after rain may be fresher, it may also be more productive. A 2012 study by Harvard Business School[9] analysed patterns in worker output and found that productivity rose significantly on rainy days. The researchers theorised that because people are less distracted by outdoor temptations, they concentrate more fully on the task at hand. A dreary afternoon, it turns out, may be the ideal time to tackle your to-do list.

MOOD-LIFTING POTENTIAL

Perhaps the most intriguing evidence of rain's effect on the body, however, lies in its ability to alter the air's electrical charge. When raindrops collide with hard surfaces – particularly during heavy downpours – they generate negative ions, which are tiny, charged particles that have long been associated with enhanced wellbeing.

Dr Michael Terman, a clinical psychologist at Columbia University in New York, discovered the mood-lifting potential of breathing in negative ions by accident. While studying the benefits of bright light therapy for seasonal affective disorder, he and his team needed a convincing placebo treatment. They turned to negative air ionisation – a method long regarded as folk science – to provide a plausible placebo. 'We fully believed it wouldn't work,' he says.

To their surprise, it did.[10] In a clinical trial, participants were divided into three groups: one received bright light therapy, one received high-density negative ion exposure, and the third received low-density ions. All were told they were being treated for winter depression. The group exposed to high-density negative ions showed significant improvements in mood over three weeks – comparable, Terman says, to people treated with antidepressants.

BUT ION THERAPY IS FREE FROM SIDE-EFFECTS

This wasn't an isolated result. Terman later saw similar improvements when testing ion therapy in patients with chronic, treatment-resistant depression, which is a very serious syndrome where there's virtually no relief from depressed mood for years at a time. It is very hard to treat with medication or psychotherapy – and yet exposure to negative ions was able to produce a statistically measurable lifting of mood. Even when testing on people without clinical depression, he found a single 30-minute exposure to negative ions helped those who experienced blue moods feel better.

There's been very little research into the mechanisms at play, but Terman has his theories: 'I like to hypothesise that inhaling negative ions may super-oxygenate the blood, mimicking the effects of aerobic exercise, and giving a mood lift,' he says.

Crucially, the level of negative ions measured after heavy rainfall is not far off the high-density levels used in Terman's studies. While more research is needed to confirm the precise links between rain, ions and mental health, the findings are certainly enough to reframe the idea of a walk in the rain. If you *are* struggling with your mental health, however, it's still important to seek support from a qualified healthcare professional.

Knowing that something beneficial is happening in the air around you after it rains – that you're breathing cleaner air, inhaling natural mood-lifters and quite possibly giving your immune system a nudge – could make going out in wet weather feel less like a trial and more like an opportunity.

So rather than resent the rain, we might be better off embracing it. A short walk, ideally in a park or woodland just after the rain has passed, could both lift your spirits and lower your stress levels, too.

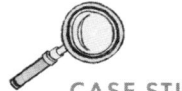

Dennis, a PhD student from Essex

'I spend most of my time indoors, and if I go for a walk, I usually do so when it's sunny, but when I tried walking in the rain I was surprised by just how amazing the scent was. It was as if the earth was giving off a sweet fragrance. Everything feels so fresh and new. I felt refreshed and invigorated afterwards.

'I've walked in the rain a few times now and I've noticed that I feel more present and chilled out. I've realised that I don't have to wait for fine weather, and I might as well make good use of the rain to get out. It seems to have improved my productivity – I feel more focused and motivated.'

HOW TO GET THE MOST OUT OF A RAINY DAY

★ **GET OUTSIDE JUST AFTER THE RAIN STOPS.** That's when the air is at its cleanest, and you'll still benefit from the petrichor as well as the ionisation in the air.

★ **GO FOR A WALK.** Even 15 minutes is enough to see benefits.

★ **BREATHE DEEPLY.** Slow, deliberate breaths through the nose can help you absorb more of the beneficial air particles.

★ **OPEN A WINDOW.** If you can't get outside, open a window after it has rained to let the fresher air in, and then breathe deeply.

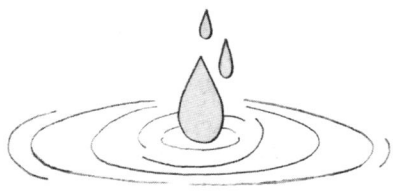

just one thing

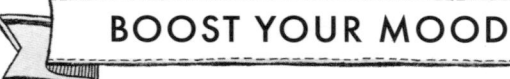

BOOST YOUR MOOD

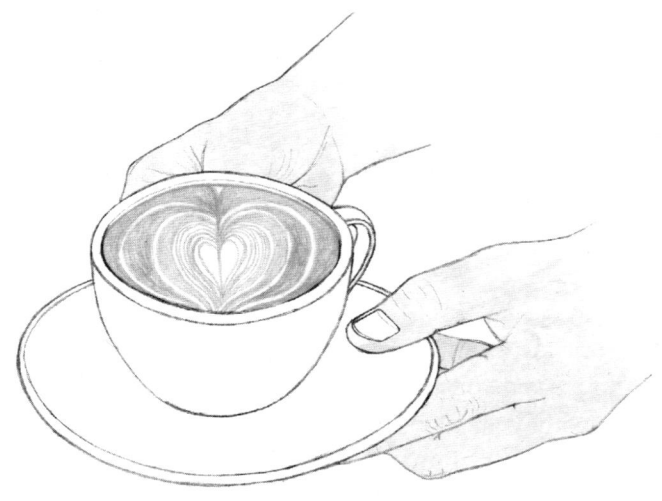

be kind

How to do it: Perform three varied acts of kindness each week.

Why do it? This may improve your mood, relieve pain and reduce chronic inflammation.

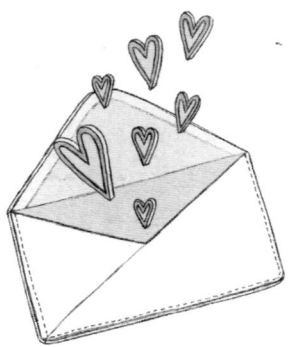

Performing a simple act of kindness isn't just a very good thing to do for someone else: studies show it could be good for you too, improving your mood, helping to relieve pain and even reducing levels of the chronic inflammation (a response by your immune system that persists long after infection or injury) that can lie behind diseases such as arthritis, cancer, heart disease and type 2 diabetes.

In fact, the science shows that even small acts of kindness, such as smiling at a stranger on the train, picking up someone else's litter or bringing in a neighbour's bins, can benefit the giver just as much as it does the receiver.

In a recent study,[11] scientists randomly allocated people with mild depression, anxiety or stress to three groups. One group performed three acts of kindness each week, the second group was asked to be more sociable and the third group tried cognitive behavioural therapy (CBT), which is known to help ease stress. After five weeks, the scientists found that acts of kindness had the greatest effect on mood, significantly reducing anxiety and depression in that group.

Brain scans show that, when someone decides to be generous or to cooperate with others, this activates a reward centre in the brain called the striatum, which normally lights up when we eat delicious food, triggering a warm glow of good feelings.

Acts of altruism also appear to have some kind of mitigating effect on the brain's perception of pain. In one rather cruel multi-part study,[12,13] volunteers were asked to donate money and were given painful electric shocks while they deliberated. Those who *did* donate reported feeling less pain. Another part of the study found the perception of pain when donating blood is less than when having blood taken for a routine test – even if the needle is twice as thick!

A 2019 study by researchers in China used MRI scans to look at brain activity and found reduced activity in parts of the brain which control pain *after* altruistic behaviour, with the effect more marked with more meaningful altruistic behaviour[14] (so you need to really feel you are being kind, and not just be going through the motions!).

REDUCES INFLAMMATION

It probably isn't too hard to imagine how a kindness mindset could lift your mood, but it is amazing to think that kindness can have a powerful effect on the immune system, by reducing inflammation and protecting your body from a host of chronic diseases, too.

Dr Tristen Inagaki is Associate Professor of Psychology at San Diego State University and has studied the way kindness can reduce the inflammatory response.[15] By testing levels of an inflammatory marker in the blood called interleukin-6 (IL-6), she was able to establish that volunteering or being kind to friends, family and organisations can effectively lower inflammation in ways that *receiving* kindness from the same people or sources does not.

This could have a dramatic impact on your health. Dr Inagaki explains: 'Systemic inflammation circulating in the blood potentially affects the whole body and leads to a host of different diseases, such as cardiovascular disease, cancer and even depression.

'Inflammation is one of the underlying mechanisms related to diseases of ageing, so it's really good to lower your levels if you can.' The more acts of kindness the better: 'A greater frequency of kindness was related to lower inflammation,' she says.

Dr Inagaki says that very large population studies support this theory by showing that kind people tend to live longer, and she believes this is probably because of the ways in which giving to others reduces subliminal perception of threat. This can help to ease stress levels, which impacts health because chronic stress has a very strong link with inflammation. 'We have evolved to have mechanisms in place to help us care for vulnerable infants in order to perpetuate the species, and now these mechanisms appear to help us care for those outside our immediate family,' she adds.

In one study,[16] Dr Inagaki and her team divided people into two groups and asked one group to write a kind, supportive note to someone in their life who might be struggling, and the other group to write a bland note about their route to work. The participants were then put through a stressful interview process involving mental arithmetic in front of a panel of judges, and their stress levels were measured throughout. Amazingly, the people who had written the kind note had a much lower physiological response to stress.

Dr Inagaki says the best way to glean the health benefits of kindness is with small but regular gestures that can fit seamlessly into your daily life. 'Maybe you can bring someone a cup of coffee or tea,' she suggests, 'bake a cake for a neighbour and leave it on their doorstep or come back from your lunch break with a drink for a work colleague.'

She says the optimal 'dose' is three acts of kindness per week – maybe one for your partner, one for another family member and one for a colleague – and she recommends varying those kind acts for maximum effect.

KINDNESS INSPIRATION

There's no limit to the number of kindness opportunities available, but if you're stuck for ideas, try these:

- ★ Compliment the first person you talk to today.

- ★ Send a positive text message to someone you haven't contacted for a while.

- ★ Smile and say 'hello' to the person next to you on the bus, on an escalator or in a shop queue.

- ★ Wave someone in front of you at the supermarket checkout if they only have a few items in their basket.

- ★ Send a 'thank you' email to someone at work who deserves more recognition.

- ★ Offer to babysit or dog walk for a neighbour.

- ★ Compliment a parent on how well behaved their child is.

- ★ Leave a post-it note for your partner telling them why you love them.

- ★ Email a former teacher who made a difference in your life.

- ★ Slow down so someone can merge in front of you in traffic.

- ★ Pick up a piece of litter and find a bin for it.

- ★ Talk to a stranger at any event who looks like they don't know anyone.

- ★ Add a positive comment to the conversation if office chatter becomes negative.

- ★ Compliment a neighbour on a feature of their home.

- ★ Call your parents or children just to say, 'I love you.'

- ★ Tell a friend what you love about their children, dog or other loved one.

- ★ Give a friend a book you think they'd like.

- ★ Forward a photo you took of a friend or their child.

just one thing

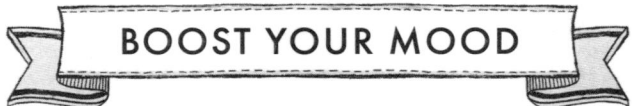

BOOST YOUR MOOD

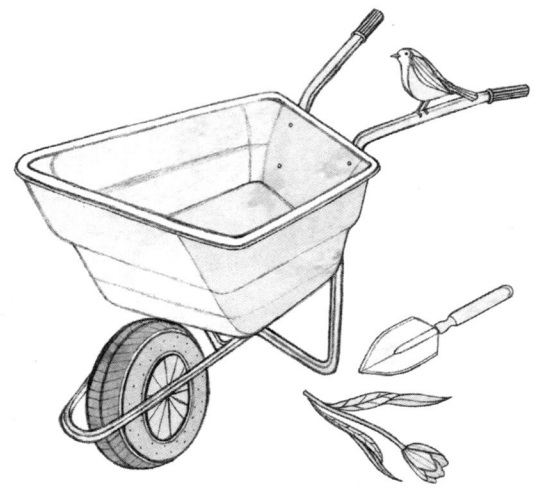

get gardening

How to do it: Do a bit of gardening.

Why do it? It may boost gut microbiome, mood, wellbeing and brain health.

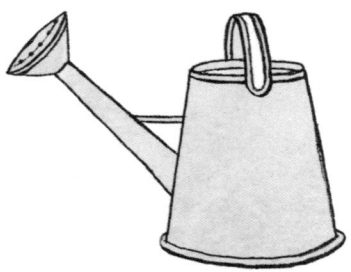

Any gardener will tell you that the physical exertion of keeping up with the digging and weeding is a great way to get fit. But you might be surprised to learn that, in addition, exposure to bacteria in soil can boost your mood and your gut microbiome. The gut microbiome is the community of micro-organisms that live in your digestive tract, playing an essential part in digestion and immune function.

There's no doubt that gardening is a great form of exercise, helping to build muscle and to reduce your risk of type 2 diabetes, which is linked with lifestyle factors and genetic predisposition. A recent study[17] of more than 140,000 Americans aged 65 and older found that the gardeners in the study were significantly less likely to have type 2 diabetes than people who engaged in other forms of exercise. This is very likely to be down to all that digging, weeding, raking and mixing fertiliser.

But as well as being good for your body, gardening is also good for your brain – and you don't need to spend long hours in the garden to reap these benefits. In one small study,[18] just 20 minutes of tending to a vegetable patch resulted in a measurable increase in levels of a hormone called BDNF (brain-derived neurotrophic factor), which has been shown to improve learning and memory. That's because, appropriately enough, BDNF acts like fertiliser for your brain cells, helping them stay in good shape. Another study has found that gardening increased levels of another important protein – VEGF (vascular endothelial growth factor), which among other things, boosts the blood supply to brain cells.[19]

TENDING TO YOUR GUT GARDEN

As our awareness of the incredibly diverse role played by our gut micro-organisms grows, studies are beginning to show that some of these health benefits occur because gardeners are unwittingly 'infecting' their digestive system with bacteria from soil.

Getting infected is generally seen as a bad thing, but some bacteria commonly found in soil look like they might be highly beneficial. For example, when lab mice were exposed to one soil bacterium called *Mycobacterium vaccae*,[20] their levels of the feel-good hormone serotonin increased. The bacterium appeared to activate neurons in areas of the brain thought to play an important role in helping animals (including humans) cope with stress.

Another study[21] found that airborne bacteria in soil dust can not only make their way into the gut microbiome of mice, but when they get there, they produce butyrate, a short-chain fatty acid which is key to keeping the gut barrier healthy.

Dr Hannah Holscher, director of the Nutrition and Human Microbiome Laboratory at the University of Illinois Urbana-Champaign, has been studying the benefits of getting your hands dirty. She has researched the ways the microbiome in our gut changes during the gardening season. 'We recruited families that gardened and families that didn't garden,' she says. 'And we asked the families to complete dietary questionnaires and to provide stool samples in late April, before the gardening season, and then again during peak gardening harvest time, in August,' she explains. 'We also collected soil samples from the gardening sites during the same time periods.'

The results were fascinating. Dr Holscher's team spotted a greater diversity of microbes in the guts of the gardening families at the end of the gardening season than the beginning. The results also showed that gardening families consume more dietary fibre than families that don't garden and have a greater microbiota diversity – specifically more of the populations of bacteria that can break down dietary fibre within the intestinal tract.

It was clear from the study that some of the microbes from the soil had made their way into the gardeners' intestinal tract. Dr Holscher says it is very likely that the bacteria were getting from the garden into the gut via the mouth. 'Perhaps it's hot, you're sweating, and a fly lands on your face and you wipe it away,' she says. 'This might mean that microscopic dirt particles are landing on your skin and potentially getting into your mouth.' Another route might be that home-grown root vegetables such as carrots or potatoes may still be covered in residual soil microbes even after they have been rinsed, she says, adding: 'There are so many different ways to be exposed to the microbes around us through touch or in our breath.'

Despite the benefits, Dr Holscher warns against eating soil on purpose: 'That would be a really bad idea,' she says. 'Gardening is great, but when you're finished, it is important to wash your hands with soap and water, and to rinse any vegetables you dig out of the garden with cold running water too.'

Previous research has shown that gardening can have a positive effect on your wellbeing, and Dr Holscher now believes that might have something to do with the way it appears to support your microbiome. Big studies of horticulture therapy for people with dementia and depression have shown that gardening can reduce stress and anxiety, and she is convinced that most people can benefit in the same way.

If you're keen to get your hands dirty, Dr Holscher recommends boosting the beneficial effects of gardening by focusing on growing healthy fruit and vegetables 'because eating the rainbow is going to provide lots of phytonutrients that have lots of different health benefits,' she says.

GARDENING FOR COMPLETE BEGINNERS

Gardening might seem out of reach if you live in a flat or have no outdoor space, but you don't need a big garden – or a garden at all – to get started. A sunny windowsill, a balcony or a few pots on a doorstep can become your green oasis. Here's how to start, even if you're a total beginner:

1. START SMALL – LITERALLY. Begin with a couple of pots or window boxes. Herbs like basil, parsley or mint are brilliant starter plants – they grow quickly, smell fantastic and are useful in the kitchen. Salad leaves, chillies and cherry tomatoes also thrive in pots.

2. USE CONTAINERS CREATIVELY. You don't need fancy planters. Old buckets, wooden crates, plastic tubs or even cut-off milk cartons can all work – just make sure they have drainage holes. Hanging baskets and vertical planters help you make the most of wall or railing space.

3. PICK THE RIGHT SPOT. Most edible plants need about six hours of sunlight a day. South- or west-facing windowsills, balconies or steps work well. If you have very little natural light, opt for shade-tolerant plants like lettuce, chard, spinach or some herbs.

4. WATER WISELY. Pots dry out quickly, so daily watering may be needed in hot weather – but don't overdo it. A good rule is to water when the top 2cm of soil feels dry. Use a saucer under pots to retain some moisture and water early in the morning or evening to reduce evaporation.

5. FEED YOUR PLANTS. Plants in pots use up nutrients quickly. A liquid plant feed (or tomato food) every couple of weeks during the growing season will keep them happy and productive.

6. BE PATIENT. Plants are forgiving, but they're also a learning curve. Some plants will die. That's okay. Keep trying.

7. JOIN THE COMMUNITY. Follow a few gardening accounts on Instagram or TikTok, preferably from your region, where the weather and soil are similar. Allotment growers and city gardeners are full of encouraging tips. You might even find a local gardening group or community project that shares seeds, advice and inspiration.

just one thing

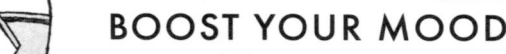

BOOST YOUR MOOD

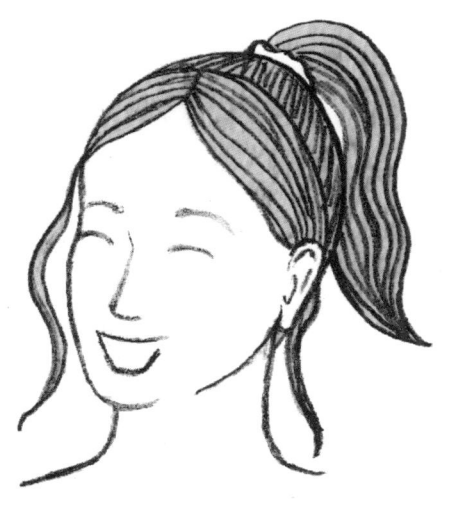

laugh out loud

How to do it: Find something (or someone) to make you laugh out loud every day.

Why do it? Laughter lifts mood and may ease pain, support memory and protect the heart.

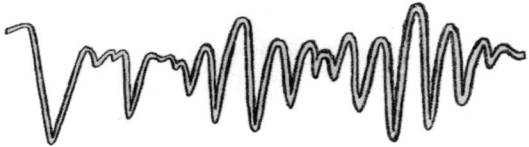

We've long known that laughter feels good. It lifts a gloomy mood, brings people together and lightens even the darkest of days. But increasingly, research suggests it does more than just boost morale – it may offer genuine health benefits.

It's perhaps no surprise that a hearty laugh triggers a cascade of physiological reactions. Laughter draws in deep gulps of oxygen-rich air, stimulates the lungs and heart, and relaxes the body. In doing so, it increases the production of endorphins – the body's natural feel-good chemicals that promote everything from pain relief to emotional connection.

There's also evidence that laughing with others is a powerful social glue. A shared chuckle builds rapport more quickly than conversation alone. Research from Oxford University[22] found that when people laugh together – say, over a clip from *Friends* or *Mr Bean* – they report stronger social bonds afterwards, even with strangers.

Intriguingly, that same study found laughter can act as a natural painkiller. Volunteers who laughed for 15 minutes at comedy videos were able to withstand 10 per cent more pain afterwards, compared with those who sat through a dry golf documentary. The belly laughers – not the mild chucklers – showed the biggest benefit, suggesting that deep, uninhibited laughter has a unique effect on the body's pain thresholds.

The power of laughter extends to the brain, too. In a small study by researchers at Loma Linda University in California,[23] older adults were shown a 20-minute comedy clip. Afterwards, they not only reported improved mood, but also performed better on memory tests. EEG (electroencephalogram) scans revealed an increase in gamma brainwave activity – a pattern associated with high-level cognitive processes like attention, learning and memory.

HEALTHY HEART

Perhaps most compelling is the evidence linking laughter to cardiovascular health. A large Japanese study[24] of over 20,000 adults found that people who reported laughing daily were 20 per cent less likely to develop heart disease compared to those who rarely laughed. Loneliness and social isolation are likely to play a role – both are known to increase cardiovascular risk – but researchers believe laughter itself may also have a direct physiological effect.

One expert who has been exploring the connection is Professor Michael Miller, a cardiologist at the University of Maryland School of Medicine in the USA. His research suggests that laughter prompts the release of nitric oxide in the bloodstream – a compound that relaxes blood vessels, lowers blood pressure, reduces inflammation and prevents the clumping of blood platelets.

'In many ways, laughter is the biological opposite of stress,' he says. 'Whereas stress causes blood vessels to constrict, laughter dilates them and sets off a cascade of protective effects.'

In one experiment,[25] Miller asked volunteers to watch two different types of film clips. One group viewed scenes from *Saving Private Ryan*, designed to induce stress. The other group watched funny films designed to elicit spontaneous laughter. The differences were marked: blood vessels in the stressed group narrowed measurably, while in the laughter group, they opened up – sometimes by as much as 50 per cent.

'Within minutes of laughing, we saw improvements in vascular function that are similar to what you'd see after aerobic exercise,' says Miller. And the mood and vascular benefits of a good belly laugh may persist for up to 24 hours – assuming nothing happens to hike your stress levels in that time.

YOU'LL LIVE LONGER, TOO

There's also early evidence that laughter may be associated with greater longevity. Centenarians consistently report a strong sense of humour and deep social networks. 'The longest-living people tend to laugh easily, often with friends, and tend to be positive,' Miller notes. 'It's hard to untangle whether laughter itself makes you live longer or whether it simply reflects a healthy outlook – but I suspect it's a bit of both.'

Miller believes we should be making laughter a deliberate part of our daily routine. 'The key to optimal heart health is to reduce stress, eat well and exercise,' he says. 'But I'd put laughter in that list too. A daily dose of humour is one of the most under-appreciated tools in the heart health toolkit.'

Fortunately, this is a prescription most of us can stick to. Whether it's watching a classic sitcom, revisiting a favourite stand-up special or simply sharing silly stories with a friend, the opportunities for laughter are plentiful – if we make space for them. A good starting point, Miller says, is to consciously seek out moments of joy. 'Find what makes you laugh and do more of it. It's not just good for your mood – it's good for your blood vessels too.'

So next time you feel a bit low, don't just power through or scroll past. Take a few minutes to watch something ridiculous, call that friend who always cracks you up or revisit a favourite comedy sketch. You'll be happy that you did!

WHAT HAPPENS TO YOUR BODY WHEN YOU LAUGH?

A proper laugh – the kind that leaves your ribs aching and your eyes streaming – triggers a full-body cascade of effects that touches almost every organ system:

1. YOUR BREATHING CHANGES. When you start to laugh, your breathing pattern changes. Air is forced out of the lungs in short bursts as the diaphragm – the muscle beneath your lungs – contracts rapidly. A deep belly laugh uses more of your respiratory system than normal breathing, increasing the intake of oxygen and boosting circulation.

2. THE HEART RATE RISES, THEN RELAXES. Initially, laughter acts like mild cardiovascular exercise: your heart rate and blood pressure may rise slightly. But soon after, they drop below your baseline, which has a calming, stress-reducing effect – much like meditation or deep breathing.

3. ENDORPHINS FLOOD THE BRAIN. Laughter prompts the release of endorphins, the brain's feel-good chemicals. These help to reduce physical pain and elevate mood. Brain imaging studies suggest that laughter activates regions involved in reward processing and social bonding.

4. MUSCLES CONTRACT AND RELAX. You may feel physically tired after a good laugh – and for good reason. Laughter activates muscles in the face, shoulders, abdomen and even legs. These contractions are followed by relaxation, which contributes to the overall sense of relief.

5. STRESS HORMONES GO DOWN. Laughter suppresses levels of cortisol and adrenaline – the body's primary stress hormones. That's why it often leaves you feeling both energised and soothed.

just
one
thing

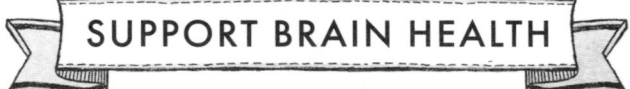

SUPPORT BRAIN HEALTH

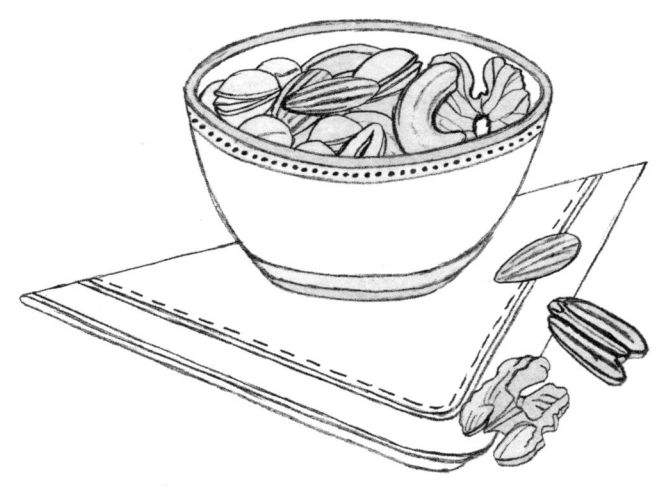

eat nuts

How to do it: Eat a small handful of unsalted nuts every day.

Why do it? This may protect against heart disease, diabetes and some cancers, while boosting brain power.

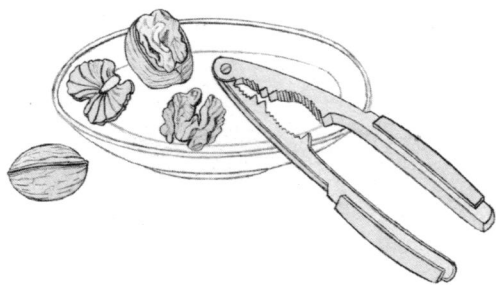

Nibbling on a small handful of nuts when you might instead have been tucking into a mid-afternoon biscuit or a chocolate treat not only means you are replacing unhealthy sugars and fats with protein and fibre, but you could also be helping to protect your heart, stave off cancer and give your brain a boost at the same time.

Nuts often get a bad press because they are high in fat, and they can cause life-threatening allergies, which is why they're rightly banned from schools and nurseries. But they are amazing little nutritional powerhouses. When we eat nuts, we get lots of fibre and, importantly, compounds called polyphenols, which feed our gut bacteria and can reduce inflammation.

Not only are the fats in nuts *healthy*, but there's some surprising new research that shows nuts can trim your waistline and even boost your brain power. In fact, it turns out making nuts a regular part of your diet could even extend your life.

The nutty thing, botanically speaking, is that most of the nuts we like to eat aren't actually nuts. Chestnuts and hazelnuts are among the only commonly eaten ones that are true nuts because they are a 'dry fruit' with a single seed encased in a hard shell. But firm favourites – almonds, cashews, pecans and walnuts – are actually classified as 'drupes' because they are seeds that develop inside a fleshy fruit. Peanuts are not technically nuts either: since they are seeds that grow in pods, they fall into the legumes category alongside beans and lentils.

All nuts are a good source of vitamin E (which protects cells against oxidative damage), magnesium (important for regulating hormones and promoting sleep), calcium (for bone health), selenium (a powerful antioxidant), copper (for healthy blood pressure) and manganese (helps regulate blood sugar). They are also high in protein, fibre and healthy unsaturated fats, and are packed with a number of compounds with antioxidant and anti-inflammatory properties, all of which are good for you. So good, in fact, that they may even help to slow the ageing process at a cellular level by protecting our 'telomeres'.

Telomeres are the caps at the end of our chromosomes (which hold our DNA). Telomeres protect chromosomes during cell division – which happens regularly to replace cells that are damaged or have reached the end of their lifespan. As we get older, telomeres gradually shrink and, when they get too short to do their job, our cells cannot divide effectively, creating many of the signs of ageing. Several studies have found a link between eating nuts and retaining the length of telomeres.[26]

Eating nuts has also been shown to reduce your risk of a whole range of diseases, including cancer, diabetes and heart disease. A Spanish study[27] of over 7,000 older adults found that people who eat nuts more than three times a week are more than 40 per cent less likely to die from cancer and 55 per cent less likely to die from heart disease compared to those who don't eat nuts. This impact was irrespective of other lifestyle factors such as alcohol consumption, physical activity and smoking.

Research from Australia also shows that eating nuts can actually give our thinking skills a boost. Dr Sze-Yen Tan works at the School of Exercise and Nutrition Sciences at Deakin University in Australia. His team published a study in 2021[28] which compared the nut intake and cognitive function of over 1,800 older adults in the USA. It found that older adults who consume nuts (a small handful of 15–30g per day) performed significantly better in terms of their short-term memory, fluency, processing speed and attention than those who didn't eat nuts.

'We found that including nuts into the diet can actually improve brain reactivity,' says Dr Tan. He believes the fatty content of nuts plays a part. The human brain is about 60 per cent fat and it needs fat in the diet to work well: 'Nuts seem to help improve the elasticity of the small blood vessels in the brain, which means there's likely to be better blood flow into the brain,' he explains.

If you're watching your weight, you might have been put off nuts because they are high in fat (about 70 per cent fat) and calories, but the fat you get in nuts is *unsaturated*, which is the sort that can actually benefit your heart health. And although nuts are pretty calorific, as long as you don't pile through too many, you won't automatically gain weight. Quite the opposite. One massive study,[29] involving more than 300,000 people, found that those who ate nuts were less likely to gain weight and had a lower risk of becoming overweight or obese.

'All the research consistently suggests that including nuts in the diet doesn't really have much effect on your body weight,' agrees Dr Tan. 'In fact, those with higher nut intake tend to have lower body weight or lower body fat percentage.'

There are a number of potential explanations for this apparent paradox. One is that we don't absorb all the fat or the energy from the nuts we consume. Another reason is that nuts make you feel full quite quickly, so a nutty snack might make you likely to eat less at the next meal. And thirdly, some studies show that we actually burn quite a lot of energy in the process of digesting nuts.

'Under a microscope, nuts are made up of lots of tiny boxes,' explains Dr Tan. 'Imagine if you have thousands of shoe boxes put together, each box contains some fat but in order to access that fat, you have to break all the shoe boxes. Chewing the nuts will break down some boxes and release the fat in them, but some boxes remain intact, and we believe around 20 per cent of fat remains inaccessible by the body.'

It is certainly worth switching out one of your daily unhealthy snacks for nuts, but don't go nuts – 15–30g a day seems to be the optimal amount. A lot of the beneficial compounds are found on the skin of the nuts, so, whether you're snacking on them or chopping them into your cooking, always aim to eat the skin too.

WHICH NUTS?

★ **ALMONDS.** *Best for: bone health and blood sugar control.* Rich in vitamin E, magnesium and calcium, almonds help maintain strong bones. They're also a source of plant protein and fibre.

★ **WALNUTS.** *Best for: brain and heart health.* These are nicknamed 'brain food' because they are the only tree nut rich in plant-based omega-3 fatty acids (ALAs), which help reduce inflammation and support heart and brain function. Walnuts also contain polyphenols with antioxidant properties.

★ **CASHEWS.** *Best for: energy metabolism and immune function.* Cashews are high in copper, which is important for energy production and brain development. They also contain zinc, which supports immunity.

★ **BRAZIL NUTS.** *Best for: thyroid support and antioxidant defence.* Brazil nuts are rich in selenium, a mineral vital for thyroid hormone production and immune health.

★ **PISTACHIOS.** *Best for: eye health and weight management.* Packed with lutein and zeaxanthin, which are antioxidants that protect eye health, pistachios also have more protein per serving than most nuts.

★ **HAZELNUTS.** *Best for: heart health and skin health.* These contain healthy monounsaturated fats, vitamin E and folate to support cardiovascular health and protect skin against oxidative stress.

★ **MACADAMIA NUTS.** *Best for: cholesterol control and anti-inflammatory benefits.* Macadamias are high in monounsaturated fats, which are linked to better heart health. They are high in calories but low in carbs.

★ **PECANS.** *Best for: cholesterol lowering and anti-inflammatory benefits.* High in antioxidants, pecans also contain compounds that may help lower LDL (low-density lipoprotein, aka 'bad') cholesterol. Pecans are a good choice for heart health.

just
one
thing

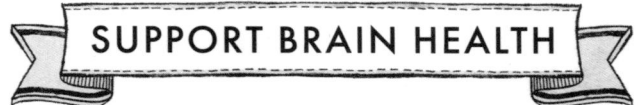

SUPPORT BRAIN HEALTH

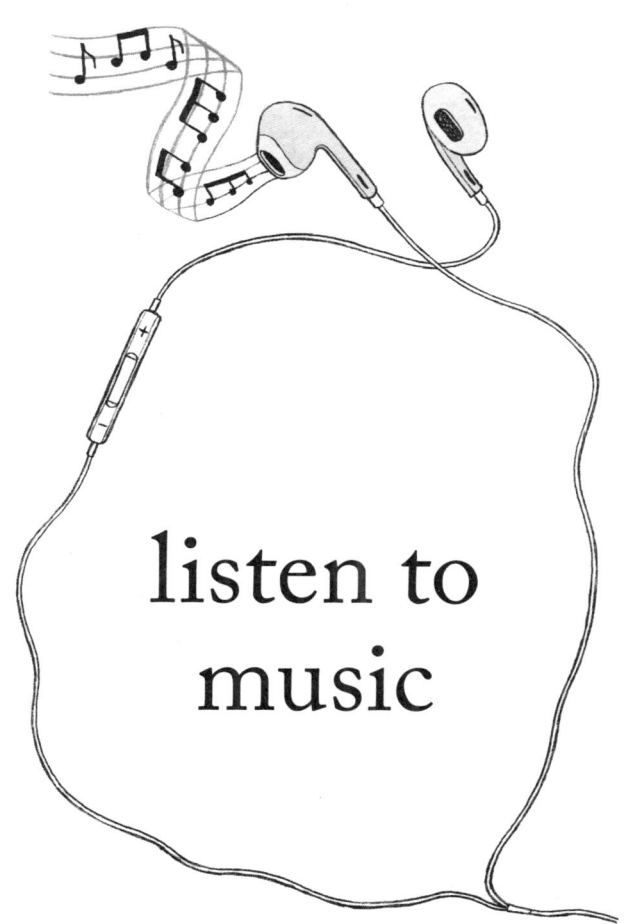

listen to
music

How to do it: Make a playlist of your favourite music and properly listen to it, without distractions, for 10 minutes each day.

Why do it? Listening mindfully to music can soothe pain, help strengthen social bonds, support cardiovascular health and bolster brain power.

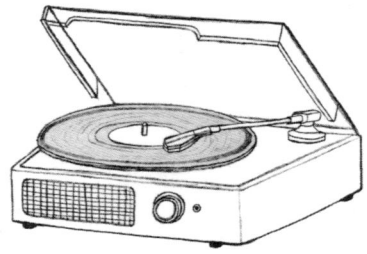

If you want a quick way to lift your spirits, put on your favourite music and really listen to it. Don't use it as background noise as you unload the dishwasher or scroll on your phone – you need to take a bit of time for proper, immersive, intentional listening.

This is a worthwhile habit to acquire, because scientists have found that listening to music – really listening – has all sorts of physical and mental benefits. It may even make you a better runner. In fact, the science of music and health is expanding in fascinating ways. One of the most intriguing findings is how music affects your blood vessels. In a small but compelling study,[30] researchers asked 10 volunteers to spend 30 minutes either listening to music they personally found joyful or listening to a standard relaxation track. The results were surprising. When participants listened to their chosen music, their blood vessels dilated significantly more than they did while listening to the relaxation track.

This widening of the blood vessels – known as vasodilation – improves circulation and allows more oxygen and nutrients to reach tissues. If it happens repeatedly over time, this kind of flexibility in the blood vessels is associated with better cardiovascular health and a lower risk of heart disease.

It turns out that the sound of good music can stimulate the brain to trigger the release of feel-good chemicals called endorphins, and also to release nitric oxide, which helps the blood vessels relax and widen.

TUNE INTO PAIN RELIEF

The endorphins released by the sound of good music have been shown to bind to opioid receptors in the brain, dampening the perception of pain and triggering a mild sense of euphoria. That's why listening to music can put a smile on your face, but it also helps to explain a growing body of research showing that music can act as a form of pain relief. Clinical trials[31] have shown that patients who listen to music as they recover from surgery require, on average, 18 per cent less morphine than those who don't have music – a significant reduction in drug use, with no adverse effects. And an extensive review of studies on music and surgical recovery[32] found patients who listened to music had a significant reduction in pain the day after surgery (needing fewer painkillers), reduced anxiety levels and lower heart rate.

TIME TO BOND

There's a curious bonding effect to be had, too. According to a study from the University of Arizona,[33] families who regularly listened to music together – in the car, at home or at concerts – reported stronger relationships later in life. Remarkably, the researchers controlled for other types of family bonding activities like eating together, playing games or going on outings, and found that music had a distinct and independent effect. One theory is that music facilitates shared emotional experiences. It also often involves synchronised movement, like tapping your feet or singing along, which releases oxytocin – the so-called 'bonding hormone' – and strengthens feelings of connection.

So playing a track everyone loves on a long drive might do more for family harmony than any lecture on gratitude ever could.

PERFORMANCE ENHANCING

There's also evidence that listening to music can improve your athletic prowess. In a treadmill study involving 30 volunteers,[34] those who listened to music during the activity were able to run longer – 15 per cent longer on average – than those without it.

It is known that playing up-tempo tracks when you're exercising helps you synchronise your movement with the rhythm, which improves efficiency and reduces the perception of exertion. In other words, it feels easier, even though you're doing the same amount of work. Selecting a slightly faster song can even trick your body into moving more quickly, because your brain naturally wants to keep time with the beat.

Dr Psyche Loui, a neuroscientist and associate professor at Northeastern University in Boston, has been using MRI scans to study precisely how listening to music alters the brain. In one of her studies,[35] healthy older adults were asked to work with music therapists to create bespoke playlists of energising and calming music. They then listened to their chosen music for one hour a day over eight weeks and kept a journal reflecting on how the music made them feel.

Before and after the intervention, the researchers conducted a battery of tests and assessments with sensors on the scalp to measure electrical activity in the brain, plus MRI (magnetic resonance imaging) scans to track blood flow to different parts of the brain in real time. The results were compelling. The scans showed regularly listening to music you love can trigger stronger communication pathways between the auditory centres of the brain (which process sound) and the reward system, the network of regions that governs motivation, emotion and pleasure.

This reward system unfortunately tends to decline in function as we get older, which can contribute to low mood, reduced motivation and cognitive sluggishness. But Loui's study suggests that listening to music might help preserve – or even restore – some of that connectivity. 'Music appears to act as a direct auditory route into these systems,' she explains. 'It stimulates learning, emotional processing and social interaction – all in one.'

Loui's team also saw measurable improvements in loneliness among participants, suggesting that music may help people feel more emotionally connected and less isolated, even when they aren't spending time with others.

When Loui and her team use a neuroimaging technique called magnetoencephalography to detect magnetic fields produced by brain activity, she says they can see the neurons almost coming alive and dancing along with the music – groups of neurons firing in time with the beat, creating a kind of internal dance.

She explains that we find this phenomenon pleasurable: 'When your brain is in sync, it is anticipating the beat, and your brain finds that rewarding and satisfying because it has guessed right!' Over time, these brain moments exercise the brain, helping to reinforce memory, support learning and maintain cognitive agility.

There's also evidence that musical 'training' like this is linked with broader cognitive benefits. Young children with musical education tend to perform better in language and mathematics tests. Older adults with musical experience not only show better working memory but are also more adept at hearing speech in noisy environments – a key factor in maintaining social interaction as we age. Recent imaging studies have shown that people with a background in music tend to have a better-connected insular cortex – a region of the brain that helps integrate emotions, bodily awareness and decision-making.

ARE YOU LISTENING CAREFULLY?

But if you really want to improve your brain's connectivity, reduce your risk of cognitive decline and boost emotional wellbeing, you need to listen to music mindfully. That means not just having music in the background but actively focusing on the sounds, the rhythms and the emotions the music evokes. By actively engaging like this, you will be stimulating not only your auditory system, but also a wide array of brain regions linked to memory, movement, reward and emotion.

The great news is that, for this process to be effective, you don't have to force yourself to listen to music you hate or just can't understand. It turns out that the most effective playlists are those you personally respond to.

One exercise used in Dr Loui's research involved creating a playlist of favourite tracks, then listening while journalling. Then try jotting down how each piece makes you feel – energised, nostalgic, calm – and what memories or thoughts it evokes. This kind of mindful listening, researchers believe, helps deepen the emotional and neurological benefits of music.

Listening to music is a free, portable, side-effect-free intervention with powerful implications for health and wellbeing. So why not press play?

A BEGINNER'S GUIDE TO MINDFUL LISTENING

Think of mindful music listening as meditation with a soundtrack. It's not about playing something in the background while you make dinner, it's about truly *hearing* the music and noticing how it makes you feel.

Start by choosing a track you love. Sit somewhere comfortable, close your eyes and listen without distractions. Let the music take up all your attention. Notice the rhythm, the instruments, the lyrics if there are any. Are there moments of tension or release? Does the music make you want to get up and move?

Try not to judge what you're hearing – there's no right or wrong response. Just observe. What emotions come up? Are there memories or images that surface? Some researchers suggest keeping a notebook and jotting down a few thoughts afterwards, which can help strengthen the brain's reward system by reinforcing positive experiences.

You can also take this practice on the move. Create a walking playlist with songs that have a strong, steady beat. Match the timing of your steps to the rhythm and allow the music to guide your pace. This can enhance both the physical and cognitive benefits of walking, while also boosting mood.

The goal is not analysis but immersion – to let music shift your inner state. As little as 10 minutes a day of focused listening can help improve memory, ease stress and deepen emotional awareness. And all it requires is a pair of headphones (or not) and your favourite tracks.

If you really want to improve your brain's connectivity, reduce your risk of cognitive decline and boost emotional wellbeing, you need to listen to music mindfully. That means actively focusing on the sounds, the rhythms and the emotions the music evokes.

just
one
thing

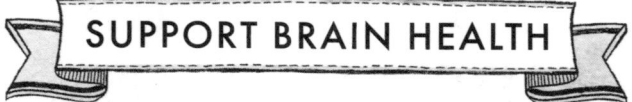

SUPPORT BRAIN HEALTH

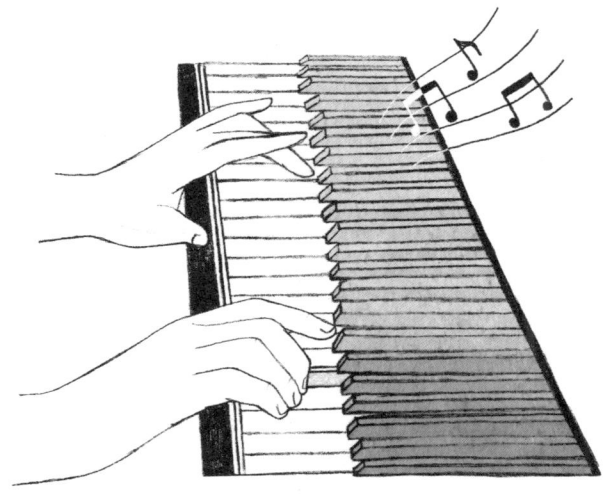

play an
instrument

How to do it: Learn to play a musical instrument.

Why do it? It may improve symptoms of depression and anxiety, and could sharpen memory, attention and motor coordination.

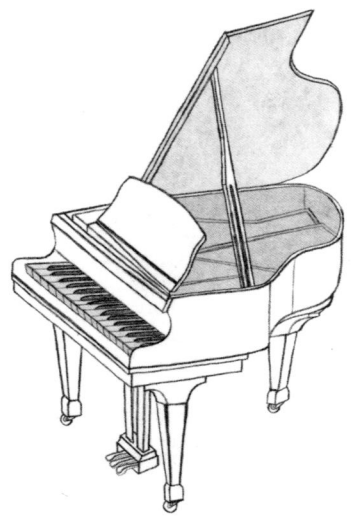

We have been making music for tens of thousands of years. In fact, one of the earliest known musical instruments is a flute made from a vulture's wing bone, thought to date back at least 40,000 years. From bone flutes to Bartók, music has been deeply woven into the story of humanity – not just as entertainment, but as a source of connection, emotion and a route to better mental and cognitive health.

Now a growing body of scientific research suggests that learning to play an instrument, even at a very basic level, can have powerful effects on our brains and bodies – particularly as we age. You don't have to be a virtuoso, or even able to play in tune. Simply engaging in musical practice has been shown to reduce symptoms of depression and anxiety, improve memory and attention, and enhance motor coordination.

In a study published in *PLOS ONE*,[36] researchers recruited 45 men and women who were receiving mental health support and randomly assigned them to one of two groups. Half were enrolled in weekly 90-minute group drumming sessions, while the others acted as a control. After 10 weeks, the drum players reported significantly reduced levels of anxiety and depression. Perhaps more impressively, these improvements were still evident three months later – long after the drumming tuition had stopped.

What set this study apart was its attempt to understand *how* drumming improved mental health. Alongside psychological questionnaires, the researchers measured inflammatory markers such as interleukin-4, which are increasingly implicated in chronic mental health conditions. They were able to show that musical intervention caused levels of inflammation to drop – but only in the group who played the drums.

'There is increasing evidence that persistent low-level inflammation contributes to conditions like depression,' says lead author Dr Daisy Fancourt of University College London. 'Music-making seems to be one of the few activities that can lower both mood symptoms and biological risk markers at the same time.'

But being actively involved in making music doesn't just lift your mood – it sharpens your senses, too. In a small study from the University of Bath,[37] researchers showed that just one hour of piano lessons a week for 11 weeks improved participants' ability to process sights and sounds. This is important for health because skills such as auditory and visual integration are crucial for everyday activities, from crossing a road to following a conversation in a noisy room.

Interestingly, the cognitive benefits of music seem to increase with age. In a study conducted in the United States,[38] older adults were randomly assigned to one of three groups: piano lessons, percussion classes or passive music listening. The active participants were asked to practise for 30 minutes a day over four months. By the end of the trial, both the piano and percussion players had improved their working memory – the system in the brain that lets you hold information temporarily and manipulate it to get things done. The piano players also saw a marked improvement in fine motor skills too, and this is key to coordination, balance and dexterity.

Dr Sofia Seinfeld, an associate professor at the Open University of Catalonia (UOC) in Barcelona, has spent much of her career investigating how musical training can preserve cognitive function in older adults. In one of her studies,[39] 20 participants aged 60–85 – none of whom had previously played an instrument – were split into two groups. One group received weekly piano lessons for four months and were encouraged to practise for at least 45 minutes a day. The control group took up other creative hobbies such as painting, computer lessons or organised sport.

At the end of the study, all participants showed some cognitive improvement, but those in the music group experienced significantly larger gains in key executive functions – including planning, attention and what's known as inhibitory control (the ability to suppress distractions or irrelevant impulses). These are vital for everyday tasks, from resisting the urge to check your phone while cooking, to managing appointments or finances.

'We also found that participants who learned an instrument showed greater improvements in mood and emotional wellbeing than those who took up painting or sport,' Dr Seinfeld says. 'Music stimulates the brain in a uniquely powerful way.'

IT'S A COMPLEX TASK

Why does music have this wide range of effects? It comes down to the complexity of the task. Reading the music, coordinating the fine motor movements required to play it, listening for mistakes and correcting them on the fly, all demand sophisticated multi-sensory processing. This activates multiple neural systems at once. When you play an instrument, your brain's auditory cortex (for processing sound), visual cortex (reading notation), motor cortex (controlling movement) and emotional centres are all simultaneously engaged.

'Music impacts brain regions related to memory, movement and emotion,' says Dr Seinfeld. 'Scans show that musicians have greater development in areas involved in auditory processing and visuospatial perception. And this can happen at any age – even if you start late in life.'

One of the most cognitively challenging aspects is learning to read music. It's essentially like learning a new language – with symbols that must be rapidly decoded and turned into precise physical movements. 'That translation process – from sight to movement to sound – is part of why music training is so beneficial,' she says. 'It pushes the brain to form new pathways.'

Crucially, music also provides its own motivation. Unlike some brain-training apps or memory drills, music is emotionally engaging. It offers a sense of progress and pleasure, which is key to maintaining any new habit. 'Even if you think you have no talent, or feel intimidated by the idea, the simple act of trying something new and challenging is hugely beneficial,' says Dr Seinfeld. 'And music has this emotional pull – people feel connected to it, which helps keep them going.'

In fact, she argues that taking up an instrument may be more effective for preserving cognitive health than some conventional brain-training methods. 'You're not just exercising your brain, you're also learning a skill that brings joy.'

The good news is that it doesn't matter which instrument you choose – or how well you play it. Whether it's a guitar, flute or keyboard, the benefits appear to be broadly similar. Nor do you need to spend a fortune. Plenty of excellent tutorials are available online for free, and many community groups offer low-cost lessons.

'You don't have to aim for concert-level proficiency,' says Dr Seinfeld. 'What matters is the engagement – the learning, the listening, the coordination. The brain doesn't care if it's Chopsticks or Chopin.' Indeed, many of the studies into music and brain health have shown significant improvements after just a few months of modest practice. Around 30 to 45 minutes a day seems to be enough to yield benefits – and consistency matters more than perfection.

If you regret not learning how to play music as a child, don't worry. In many ways, adults may be better learners because they have stronger discipline, more patience and clearer goals.

just
one
thing

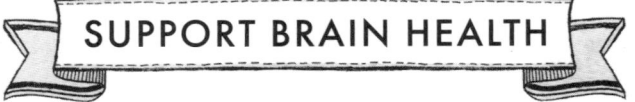

SUPPORT BRAIN HEALTH

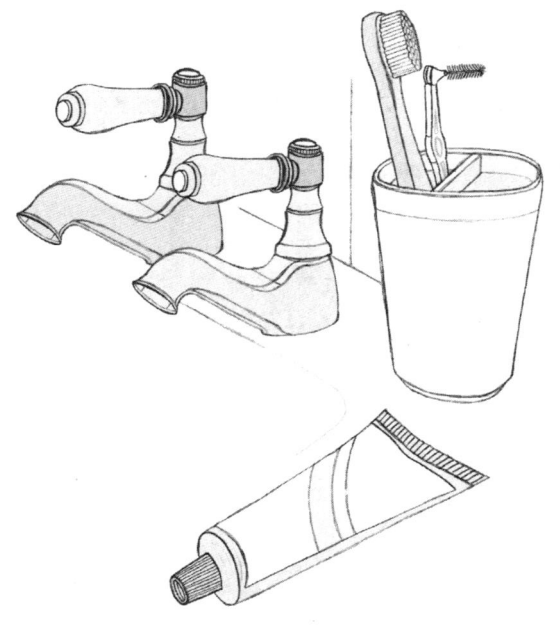

look after
your teeth

How to do it: Brush your teeth twice a day and also use floss or interdental brushes.

Why do it? It may reduce your risk of heart disease, stroke and dementia.

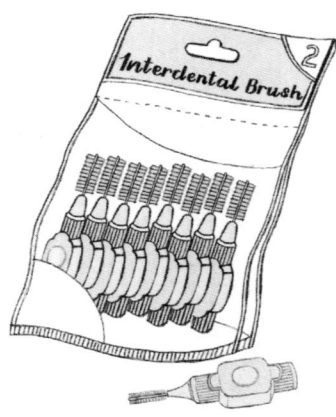

We all know it's a very good idea – for the health of our teeth and gums – to brush our teeth twice a day, but emerging research indicates there may be many more surprising health benefits to be had from making a point of keeping your pearly whites sparkling.

Surprisingly, in the UK, a quarter of all adults don't brush their teeth twice a day. And when it comes to men, it is one in three who don't. It turns out those slack-brushers might be making a big mistake because good dental hygiene doesn't just prevent cavities and freshen your breath, it could also reduce your risk of stroke, stave off dementia and protect multiple aspects of your health.

Dr Sim Singhrao from the University of Central Lancashire School of Dentistry explains that poor or infrequent brushing can lead to gum disease: 'Dental plaque and bacteria become wedged between the gum and the enamel and form pockets,' she says. 'If left like that, this eventually erodes the soft tissues and even the hard tissues, leading to bleeding – and ultimately your teeth will fall out.'

If that's not bad enough, scientists now know that the bacteria from your bleeding gums can enter the bloodstream and travel throughout the body. This activates an immune response that can lead to chronic inflammation, which damages the inner lining of your blood vessels, increasing fatty build-up, which in turn can affect blood flow to your vital organs. 'We now know that conditions such as type 2 diabetes, arthritis, cardiovascular diseases and stroke can all be related to gum disease,' says Dr Singhrao. 'Although some bacteria in your mouth are helpful, the ones that cause gum disease can affect your whole body, causing damage to organs far away from your mouth,' she explains.

That's why anything you can do to prevent the build-up of bacteria in your gums will not only save your teeth but could potentially provide significant long-term health benefits. For example, studies show that keeping your gums in good shape can benefit your heart. According to a huge study conducted on over 10,000 men and women from the Scottish Health Survey,[40] people who brush their teeth twice a day have lower rates of heart disease than those who brush once a day or less.

Poor dental hygiene clearly impacts your immune system. One review of studies[41] found that in people with severe gum disease, immune cells called neutrophils were overactivated, potentially weakening the body's ability to fight infections elsewhere. Another big review of trials[42] found that treating gum disease led to measurable reductions in markers of systemic inflammation, such as C-reactive protein, which is often elevated when the immune system is under strain.

Another really good reason for keeping your teeth and gums in good shape is because doing so may also protect your brain. A study of stroke patients[43] revealed that over 80 per cent had blood clots that contained the microscopic presence of oral bacteria. And other studies[44] show that people who have inflamed gums are also at greater risk of Alzheimer's disease.

Dr Singhrao was among the first to prove the way that bacteria cross the blood–brain barrier to get into your brain. Her team compared brain tissue from people diagnosed with Alzheimer's disease and tissue from a healthy brain – and found DNA from gum bacteria exclusively in the Alzheimer's brains.

TOOTH CARE

Not surprisingly, Dr Singhrao strongly advises we all brush our teeth twice a day for at least two minutes each time, first thing in the morning and last thing at night. She also suggests using a fluoride toothpaste to brush your teeth and not finishing with a rinse, so that you can allow some of the toothpaste to linger on your teeth and gums to give added protection. 'We were surprised to find in our research that the tongue gets very dirty too, so it is important to clean your tongue when you're brushing,' she adds.

Regular visits to the dentist are certainly a very good idea. If you have healthy teeth and gums, you can probably get away with going every 12–24 months, but your dentist may prefer to see you every 6 months if you have diabetes, a weakened immune system or a history of cavities or gum disease.

Listen to your dentist's advice, but most of us would also benefit from flossing or using interdental brushes to get to those tricky-to-reach bits, but it's best to floss *before* you brush your teeth, not after. A study of dental students in Iran[45] found that flossing before rather than after brushing removed the most plaque. That's because floss or interdental brushes loosen and dislodge plaque and food particles from between the teeth and below the gumline, making it easier for the toothbrush to effectively clean those areas. It also means the fluoride in your toothpaste gets to reach more of your tooth surface, so maximising its protective benefits.

Another tip from the British Dental Association is to brush your teeth before breakfast – not after – and to wait a full hour after your evening meal before you start your night-time brushing routine again. That's because eating creates acid in the mouth which can weaken your enamel, so brushing too soon after a meal could actually damage your teeth.

ELECTRIC TOOTHBRUSHES: THE SMARTER CHOICE FOR CLEANER TEETH

Swapping your manual brush for an electric one could do more than just simplify brushing – it may significantly boost oral health. A 2014 Cochrane review,[46] summarising over 5,000 participants, found electric models reduce plaque by up to 21 per cent and gum inflammation by around 11 per cent, compared with manual toothbrushes after three months.

The advantage becomes even more pronounced with modern oscillating-rotating brushes. A clinical trial[47] involving 110 adults showed that, after eight weeks, 82 per cent of electric-brush users achieved healthy gum scores, compared to just 24 per cent with manual brushes – a 14.5-fold increase. And in children, oscillating electric models reduced back-of-mouth plaque by over 108 per cent, outperforming manual brushes in every measured area.[48]

Sonic and oscillating brushes both deliver results, and dentists note that, while technique and consistency are key, electric brushes do much of the work for the user. Features like built-in timers, pressure sensors and multiple brushing modes also ensure users stick to the recommended two minutes and avoid damaging enamel – benefits particularly suited to those with limited dexterity or braces.

So an electric toothbrush might be a wise long-term investment in oral health. You can save money by buying one handset for the family, plus a fresh brush head for everyone who uses it.

CHEWING GUM

You can boost your oral health and reduce your risk of tooth decay by chewing sugar-free gum after meals. A 2020 meta-analysis study[49] found that regular use of sugar-free gum led to a 28 per cent reduction in the development of dental cavities, rising to 33 per cent when the gum was sweetened with xylitol alone.

The key lies in the way gum increases saliva production, which neutralises harmful acids, helps wash away food particles and supports enamel remineralisation. Xylitol, a naturally derived sweetener used in many gums, has also been shown to slow down the growth of Streptococcus mutans, the bacteria primarily responsible for cavities.

While dentists still stress that chewing gum is no substitute for brushing and flossing, it can be a useful addition to a daily oral-care routine.

just
one
thing

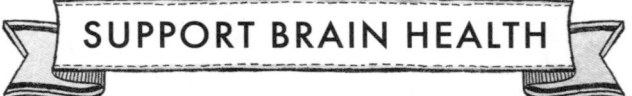

SUPPORT BRAIN HEALTH

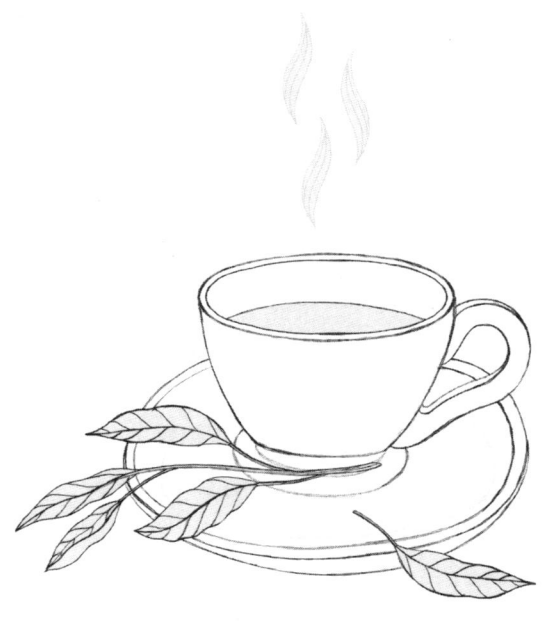

drink green tea

How to do it: Drink three cups of green tea every day.

Why do it? It may improve mood and heart health, while protecting the brain from cognitive decline.

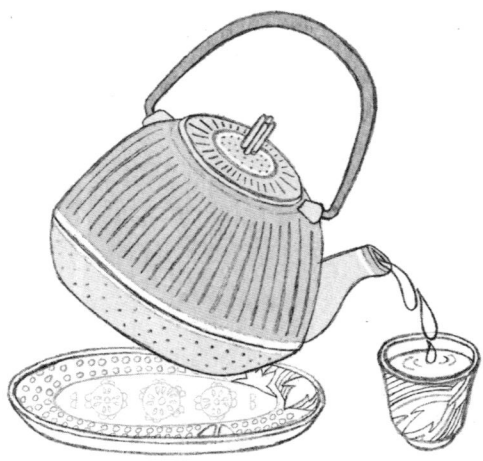

There are plenty of health benefits to be had from drinking a cup of ordinary tea or coffee (as long as you don't stir in too much milk and sugar), as you can read on pages 107–11, but emerging research shows that green tea could have extra special benefits for brain health and wellbeing. In fact, a regular green tea habit could help to improve your mood, your heart health and even protect your brain from cognitive decline.

Green tea has a tangy bitterness to it – a distinct flavour that comes from the high levels of antioxidant polyphenols that provide its potency. One of these polyphenols, a hard-to-pronounce molecule called epigallocatechin gallate (EGCG), lies behind many of the purported health benefits, from helping you burn more fat to breaking down harmful plaques in your blood vessels – and even potentially staving off diseases such as dementia.

Scientists at the University of Leeds believe drinking green tea could reduce your risk of heart attack or stroke. Their studies[50] have shown that EGCG can bind to and break up potentially dangerous plaques in your blood vessels.

Other studies have shown that compounds in green tea may also help you burn more visceral fat – the fat that accumulates inside your organs and which has been linked to chronic illnesses such as heart disease and type 2 diabetes. In one small study,[51] people who took a green tea extract before exercising burned 17 per cent more abdominal fat than those who didn't take the supplement. One theory is that green tea may increase the number of mitochondria, the powerhouses in your cells, which in turn could increase your energy expenditure. More mitochondria equals more energy burn.

DEMENTIA PROTECTION

But perhaps more surprisingly, there's research which suggests that this one polyphenol in green tea, EGCG, which isn't in ordinary black tea, can boost your brain power and may even protect your brain from diseases like dementia.

Dr Edward Okello from the University of Newcastle has been researching the impact of green tea on the brain. He believes the EGCG in green tea effectively increases levels of a brain chemical called acetylcholine, which in turn increases a process called 'neurotransmission' (the transfer of information between neurons), which translates into improved cognitive function.

He explains that, as we get older, the chemical activity that enables us to react to internal and external stimuli, recall information in both short and long term, and access memories, naturally declines. The chemical activity is facilitated by acetylcholine, levels of which naturally decline as we age. 'They decline faster if you succumb to a disease like dementia of the Alzheimer's type,' he says.

Acetylcholine is naturally recycled or broken down by an enzyme called acetylcholine esterase, but Dr Okello's studies show EGCG can slow down the action of this enzyme, so effectively boosting levels of acetylcholine and protecting the brain from rapid decline.

He and his team have also researched the impact of consuming green tea on a protein called amyloid, which is one of the drivers of dementia. 'Amyloid proteins can aggregate and form plaques in the brain, which are quite destructive to our brain cells and affect our cognition,' he says. He explains that green tea has a protective effect on an enzyme called beta-secretase, which helps to break down the amyloid precursor protein, so preventing it from forming those destructive plaques. He believes that drinking green tea could help you prevent or at least delay the build-up of amyloid in the brain.

Although this research is mostly based on animal studies, human studies which analysed the amyloid build-up in the spinal cord after drinking green tea show that the tea helps to clear the amyloid load in the system. One of Dr Okello's studies[52] looked at green tea consumption in people aged 85-plus over a six-year period. It showed that green tea consumption slows cognitive decline over time.

Dr Okello has published a pilot study[53] that assessed electrical activity in the brain after green tea consumption and found that it enhanced alpha, beta and theta brainwaves. Alpha waves are associated with relaxed alertness, beta waves with focused thinking and active concentration, and theta waves with gentle, meditative attention. Together, these shifts suggest green tea promotes a unique mental state of calm focus.

This, he says, means that green tea can help fulfil the dual function of making you feel both relaxed and alert, as well as able to concentrate better without overstimulation. His researchers were able to see healthy, de-stressing changes in brainwave activity.

One reason could be the way EGCG works with the caffeine in green tea and an amino acid called L-theanine, which gives ordinary black tea its calming and relaxing effects. The EGCG has a calming action, while L-theanine increases a chemical called gamma-aminobutyric acid (GABA) in the brain, which can help slow down brain activity, making you feel calmer and more at ease.

For the studies, the researchers brewed green tea, then freeze-dried it to create a powder so they could accurately calculate the amount of EGCG being delivered. This is similar to the process used to create matcha (see the box below), which has two or three times as much EGCG per cup than a standard brewed cup of green tea.

But Dr Okello believes that drinking at least three cups of green tea a day would have a similar effect and certainly be preferable to taking green tea supplements, which usually contain other components that may compromise the activity of the tea.

HOW TO BREW THE PERFECT CUP OF GREEN TEA

If you don't like the bitter taste of green tea, try using cooler water. The process of boiling water releases tannins, which give the bitter taste. If you have a kettle with temperature control, set it to 79–85°C. If you're using a regular kettle, let the boiled water cool for a minute, or pour between two containers to accelerate the cooling.

Although tea bags of green tea work well, Dr Okello recommends buying loose tea, because it diffuses more easily in hot water. 'Use a tea diffuser and steep the leaves in the hot water for three minutes,' he suggests.

You'll find green tea in any supermarket, either alone or blended with other herbs and spices. Jasmine flowers, for instance, add fragrant volatile oils that have been linked to relaxation and reduced heart rate; ginger will give an additional anti-nausea effect; and peppermint is known to aid digestion.

WHAT'S MATCHA?

Matcha is a type of green tea – but with a notable difference in how it's grown, processed and consumed. It is made from the leaves of the *Camellia sinensis* plant, just like all traditional green teas. However, about three weeks before harvest, matcha tea plants are shaded from direct sunlight. This triggers an increase in chlorophyll and the amino acid L-theanine, giving matcha its vivid green colour and distinctive umami flavour.

Once harvested, the leaves are steamed, dried and ground into a fine powder. Unlike regular green tea, matcha powder is whisked directly into hot water – so you consume the whole leaf.

This difference in preparation means matcha delivers a more concentrated dose of nutrients. It tends to be higher in antioxidants, particularly EGCG (epigallocatechin gallate), and provides a more sustained release of caffeine due to the presence of L-theanine, which moderates energy and promotes calm alertness.

just
one
thing

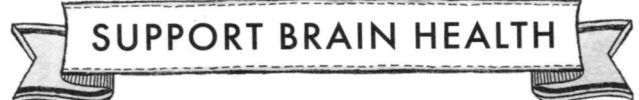

SUPPORT BRAIN HEALTH

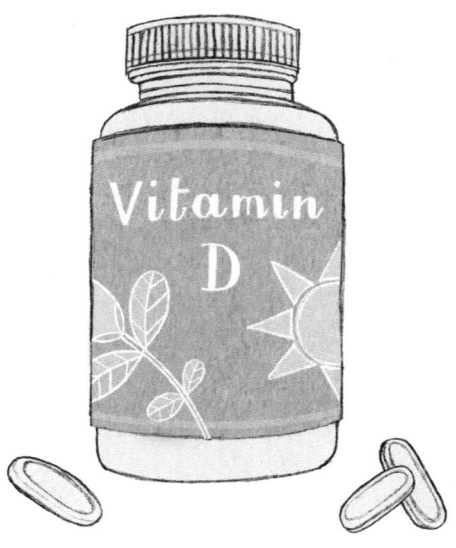

take vitamin D

How to do it: Take a 10mcg vitamin D tablet every day in the winter months.

Why do it? It may offer immunity support, inflammation control, mood regulation and protection from dementia.

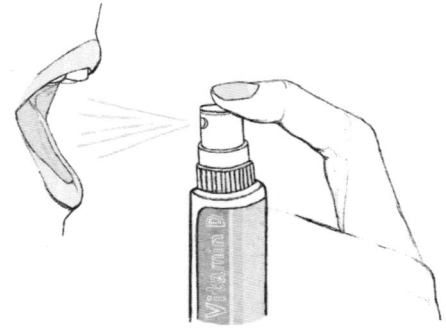

During the summer months, most of us can keep our vitamin D levels topped up with regular sun exposure and a little oily fish in the diet. But by autumn, those stores will have dwindled, and during the long UK winter months, deficiency can emerge as a serious health concern.

Vitamin D is well known for being good for our bones, but it's not just our bones that pay the price if we don't get enough of it. New research shows that low vitamin D can undermine immunity, mood, inflammation control – and potentially even speed cognitive decline.

Ideally, everyone should take a daily 10mcg (400 IU) supplement during winter. In fact, this is now the NHS recommendation. Though slight, this dose is enough to raise levels into a healthy range for most people.

Since its discovery in the 1920s, vitamin D's role in calcium absorption and bone health has been well understood. Its recorded triumph over rickets is well documented. However, the recent discovery of vitamin D receptors across virtually all body tissues suggests effects far beyond bone.

From March to October, the UVB rays we get from sunshine in the UK are, for most of us, strong enough. Just 10 to 15 minutes of sun exposure on the arms and face a few times a week in summer can often generate enough vitamin D – but this varies depending on your skin type and other factors. Dietary sources – fatty fish and eggs – are useful but they contribute only small additional amounts. However, a 10mcg daily supplement is particularly a good idea if you are elderly, if you don't get much sun exposure, if you have a darker skin tone or you are at risk of fragility.

FEWER COLDS

Vitamin D's impact on infection is clear: it supports the activation of T-cells, which are immune cells that protect the body from infection, and it also helps to regulate the immune response to reduce the risk of chronic inflammation afterwards. Studies consistently show supplementation reduces the number of colds you get and can shorten the duration of symptoms. It does this by enhancing the activity of immune cells such as macrophages, which engulf and destroy pathogens, and also by stimulating the production of antibiotic-like proteins (defensins) that protect the respiratory tract.

BRAIN SUPPORT

Vitamin D's role in mood was recently confirmed by a big meta-analysis of over 40 randomised controlled trials. The analysis found that higher doses – 5–10 times the standard 10mcg (400 IU) – can alleviate depressive symptoms.[54]

Everyday supplements might offer much lower doses, but the speculation is that they can help to protect against seasonal dips in mood. This thinking is aligned with the relatively recent discovery of vitamin D receptors in the prefrontal cortex, the brain's emotional control centre.

An emerging link between vitamin D and cognitive decline is drawing considerable interest. Professor David Llewellyn of Exeter University was able to use US population data to reveal that vitamin D deficiency increases Alzheimer's risk by 50 per cent, and full-blown vitamin D deficiency could raise dementia risk by 125 per cent.[55] Genetic studies support these observational trends. 'There are multiple mechanisms at play,' he explains. 'Vitamin D does seem to interact with the clumps of abnormal protein, amyloid plaques and tau in the brain, which are the hallmarks of Alzheimer's disease. Normally these clumps are difficult to break down, but vitamin D seems to help with cleaving or chopping up these abnormal proteins and clearing them from the brain.'

Other scientists have argued that vitamin D helps to protect the blood supply to the brain and reduce inflammation, which might make it useful for other types of dementia. The jury is still out on this one. A 2024 trial in the USA found giving older adults a high-dose supplement of vitamin D had a minimal effect on reducing dementia incidence, although the impact was more apparent in those with darker skins, who tend to have lower baseline vitamin D levels.[56] However, a recent UK Biobank analysis[57] observed that regular supplement use by mid-life adults (aged 55–69) lowered Alzheimer's risk by 17 per cent and vascular dementia by 14 per cent.

These findings are observational and cannot prove causation, but they underline a consistent pattern: people who take vitamin D supplements regularly tend to have lower dementia risk.

SLOWING THE AGEING PROCESS

There are very new reports from epidemiology centres[58] which suggest that very high vitamin D supplementation – at least 2,000 IU per day – slightly slows cellular ageing by preserving the length of telomeres. These structures (which protect our chromosomes, which hold our DNA) naturally shorten as we get older – and this shortening is linked to many age-related conditions such as cardiovascular disease, diabetes and some cancers.

But large doses of vitamin D are not recommended in the general population. And individuals on certain medications – including steroids, anti-epileptics or diuretics – should speak to their doctor before taking a supplement.

Official NHS guidance now recommends a daily 10mcg supplement for all from October to March – including children, pregnant women, housebound adults and those with darker skin or limited sun exposure. Certainly, UK observational studies point to modest reductions in blood pressure and inflammation (marked by C-reactive protein) in older adults taking standard supplements.

While major trials continue, including international dementia studies, it seems sensible to top up your vitamin D in the winter months. It's not a wonder drug, but it is a profoundly important foundation for health. In the gloom of winter, it's a small tablet with a big promise.

HOW TO CHOOSE A VITAMIN D SUPPLEMENT

When selecting a vitamin D supplement, experts recommend looking for clarity on dosage, absorption and quality. There are two main forms of vitamin D: D2 (ergocalciferol) and D3 (cholecalciferol). Studies show that D3 is more effective at raising blood levels of vitamin D, so most experts advise choosing a supplement that contains D3. For vegans, plant-based D3 derived from lichen is now widely available.

Absorption matters, too. Vitamin D is fat-soluble, meaning that it's best taken with a meal containing healthy fats (such as nuts or olive oil). Some formulations suspend D3 in oil (such as olive or coconut) to improve uptake – these may be particularly helpful for people with digestive issues.

Liquid drops allow flexible dosing and are especially useful for infants, children and those with difficulty swallowing pills. Chewable tablets and gummies are popular with children and adults who prefer a more palatable option, though they may contain added sugars. Sprays deliver vitamin D directly into the mouth for rapid absorption via the oral mucosa, which can be helpful for individuals with digestive issues, too.

Do check the supplement you choose is third-party tested or approved by a reputable body such as the UK's Medicines and Healthcare products Regulatory Agency (MHRA). This helps ensure it contains the stated dose and is free from contaminants.

HOW DO WE MAKE OUR OWN VITAMIN D FROM SUNSHINE?

When ultraviolet B (UVB) rays from sunlight hit your bare skin, a chemical reaction occurs in the epidermis, the outermost layer: UVB light converts a cholesterol-based compound in your skin called 7-dehydrocholesterol into vitamin D3 (cholecalciferol).

This vitamin D3 is then transported to the liver, where it's converted into calcidiol, the storage form. From there, the kidneys (and some other tissues) convert it into calcitriol, the active form of vitamin D, which the body can use.

This process is influenced by:

★ **SKIN COLOUR.** Darker skin has more melanin, which blocks UVB and slows vitamin D production.

★ **TIME OF DAY.** Midday sunlight contains the most UVB.

★ **SEASON AND LATITUDE.** In the UK, from October to March, sunlight is too weak to make much vitamin D.

★ **SUNSCREEN AND CLOTHING.** These block UVB rays, reducing production, which is why many doctors recommend allowing yourself 15 minutes of sun exposure before applying sunscreen (as long as you don't burn in that time) and rolling up your sleeves to expose your skin to the sun when it is safe to do so.

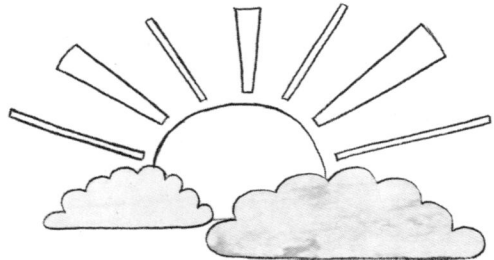

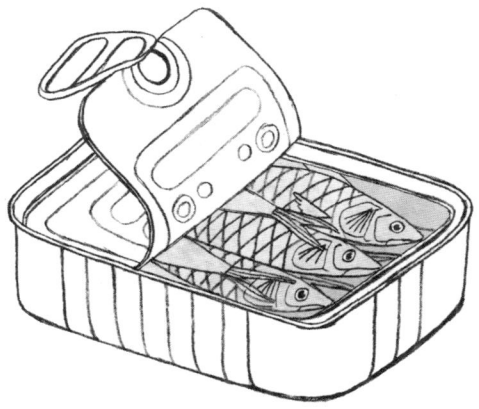

TOP FOOD SOURCES OF VITAMIN D

Vitamin D is notoriously hard to obtain from diet alone, but food can provide a useful supplement, particularly in the winter months:

★ The best natural source is oily fish such as salmon, mackerel, sardines and trout. A single portion of cooked salmon can provide more than half the recommended daily intake. Cod liver oil is another concentrated source.

★ Egg yolks also contain small amounts of vitamin D, as do liver and red meat.

★ Fortified foods play a key role: many brands of breakfast cereal, plant-based milks (like soya or oat) and some dairy products are enriched with added vitamin D. Look for 'fortified with vitamin D' on the packaging. For vegetarians and vegans, fortified foods and supplements are often the most reliable options.

★ Some mushrooms – particularly those exposed to UV light – can also offer modest amounts of vitamin D.

just
one
thing

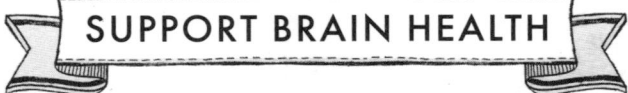

SUPPORT BRAIN HEALTH

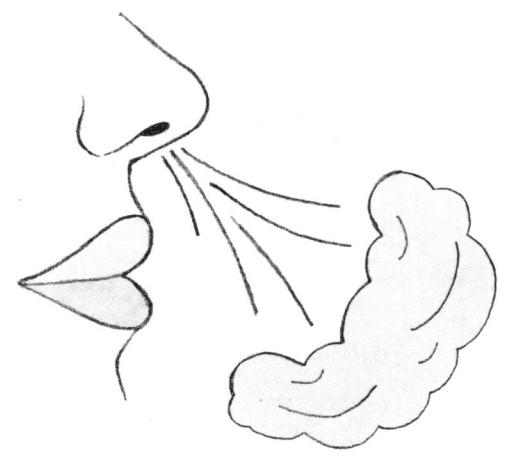

breathe through your nose

How to do it: Keep your lips closed and breathe through your nose!

Why do it? It could increase oxygen uptake and improve gum health, immunity and memory.

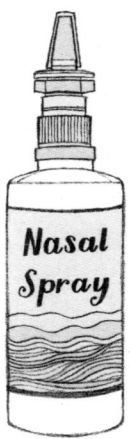

It seems ridiculously simple but making a conscious effort to breathe in through your nose could benefit your health more than taking a handful of supplements. The science is surprisingly clear: this small shift in behaviour could be enough to increase your oxygen uptake, help you maintain gum health, strengthen your body's immune response and possibly even sharpen your memory.

That's because nasal breathing changes the way air enters and interacts with the body. When you inhale through your nose, the air is filtered, humidified and warmed before it reaches your lungs. It turns out that this process is key to improving lung function and protecting respiratory health. It also appears to influence blood flow and, intriguingly, seems to enhance cognitive function, too.

At the very least, remembering to breathe through your nose will keep your mouth healthier. When your nose is bunged up with a cold and you have to breathe through your mouth for a protracted period, you might notice that you can end up with a dry mouth. This is caused by reduced stimulus to the salivary glands and by water evaporating from saliva, reducing saliva flow. This drying effect disrupts the oral microbiome and impairs the mouth's natural defences, which can lead to tooth decay and gum inflammation. In fact, dentists regularly note that chronic mouth breathers are more prone to dental problems.

Perhaps more importantly, it seems nose breathing may even give your brain a boost. In one study,[59] volunteers were put into a brain scanner and given challenging memory tasks. Their performance improved significantly when they breathed through their noses compared to when they used their mouths. The scans showed the brains of the nose breathers were working more efficiently, with heightened activity in parts of the brain related to memory and attention.

Spatial awareness is affected, too. This is the ability to perceive and interact with the environment. In Israel, researchers monitored brainwaves while volunteers manipulated 3D shapes.[60] They found that each nasal inhalation was accompanied by increased brain activity in areas associated with spatial reasoning. Participants also performed their tasks more accurately when breathing through their noses.

It is worth noting that, in contrast, exhaling through the mouth can be beneficial in certain situations, such as during physical exertion or when practising specific breathing techniques.

WHY IT WORKS

Scientists now believe that the remarkable effects of nose breathing could be explained by the presence of a gas called nitric oxide (NO). This gas plays a crucial role in regulating cardiovascular function by dilating blood vessels and easing blood flow. It also helps reduce blood pressure. At higher concentrations, NO has antimicrobial properties, helping the body fight off infections.

The body produces NO naturally, and because it can be detected on the breath, until relatively recently it was thought this gas was produced in the lungs. However, Professor Jon Lundberg of the Karolinska Institute in Sweden was among the first to discover that it is actually the nasal cavities that produce nitric oxide in meaningful quantities.

The discovery, he recalls, was accidental. 'We were in the lab measuring the small amounts of nitric oxide being produced by volunteers,' he explains. 'But one of the volunteers felt uncomfortable breathing through his mouth and switched to nose breathing. We put a face mask on him to catch the NO and suddenly the readings went sky high – two to five times more of the gas was being produced. That's when we realised NO was being generated in the nose and being drawn into the lungs – and not being generated in the lungs at all.'

This discovery helps explain the sterile nature of the sinuses in healthy people, even when the nasal cavity is full of bacteria. 'The high concentration of NO in the sinuses probably helps to sterilise them,' says Lundberg.

The second effect is even more intriguing. When NO reaches the lungs it helps to dilate blood vessels, particularly in the upper regions of the lungs, where blood flow is typically poor due to the effects of gravity. The more NO the better. 'Better blood flow means more efficient oxygen uptake,' says Lundberg. 'And oxygen is essential to nearly every bodily process, from brain function to immune response.'

Circulation improved by healthy NO production could also help the lungs defend against infection, he explains: 'In areas with poor blood flow, pathogens are more likely to take hold, which is why diseases like tuberculosis often affect the upper lungs.' His studies[61] showed a 25 per cent increase in blood flow to these areas when people inhaled through the nose, and he is convinced that change was driven entirely by NO. By redistributing blood flow, nasal breathing supports the lungs' natural defences, he says, although levels of NO that reach the lungs are too low to have a strong antimicrobial effect.

UNLOCKING THE POWER OF NASAL BREATHING

Professor Lundberg suggests the first step to begin reaping these benefits is to become aware of your daily breathing patterns. Work out whether you are typically a nose or a mouth breather and aim to spend more time breathing through your nose.

Of course, not everyone finds nasal breathing easy. Chronic allergies, sinus infections or nasal blockages can make it difficult or even impossible. But if there's nothing structurally wrong with your nose, consciously thinking about breathing through your nose is a simple and effective way to support your overall health and wellbeing. Here are some tips for getting started:

1. CLEAR YOUR NOSTRILS. If you're someone who struggles with nasal breathing due to congestion, try using a saltwater spray to clear the nostrils.

2. CLOSE YOUR LIPS. Try to keep your lips gently closed except when talking, eating or exercising vigorously. If you find it tricky, start with just 10 minutes at a time. Then build to doing it when walking or doing light exercise. If necessary, set a reminder on your phone – if you've always breathed through your mouth, it's easy to slip back into mouth breathing without noticing.

3. TAPE YOUR LIPS. When nasal breathing becomes familiar, try taping your mouth shut for short periods during the day. Use sensitive skin medical tape (such as Micropore) or specially designed mouth strips. Apply the tape vertically in the centre of your lips so you can still breathe or speak. Start by wearing tape for 10–30 minutes, then build to taping during short naps or the first hour of sleep. If you tolerate partial sealing well, you can try a horizontal strip across your lips, but don't try this if you have severe nasal congestion, sleep apnoea or breathing difficulties.

4. TRY HUMMING. Humming, it turns out, isn't just relaxing. Five to ten seconds of humming is enough to flush out the sinuses and give the immune system a boost. That's because humming generates oscillating sound waves that pass through the tiny openings connecting the nasal cavity to the sinuses. These vibrations create turbulence that helps ventilate the sinuses. In fact, studies[62] have shown that just one short bout of humming can completely exchange the air in the sinuses – a process that otherwise takes five to six hours of normal breathing.

just
one
thing

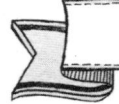

REDUCE STRESS

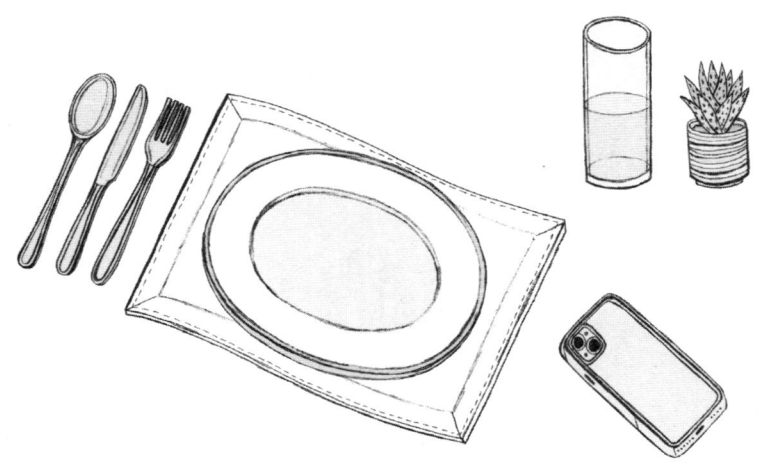

use your mobile
phone less

How to do it: Reduce your mobile phone use by one hour a day.

Why do it? This may reduce stress, improve mood and cognition, enhance social life and relationships – and even enhance your posture.

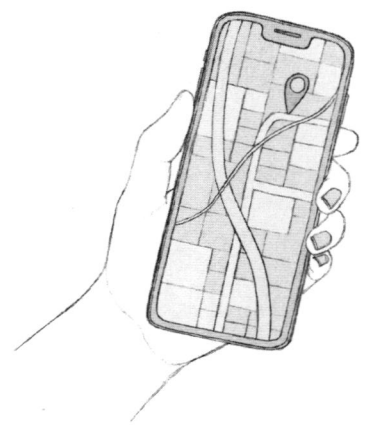

Although smartphones are very clever and undoubtedly useful (it's great to find instant answers to queries or to navigate with ease around a new city), they do have a negative side. Studies show that the time we spend engrossed with and distracted by these pocket-sized computers can interfere with our sleep, our mood and our productivity.

Over 90 per cent of UK adults own a smartphone. And it is claimed that, worldwide, there are now more mobile phones than toothbrushes. And most of us don't just use that phone for chatting – it's likely to be our diary, our encyclopaedia, our navigator, our camera and a cherished source of entertainment.

It's no surprise that we can become worryingly addicted. In the UK, we spend an average of four hours a day online, three of which are on the phone, and more than two hours on social media. In fact, statistics show that most of us check our phones

58 times a day on average.[63] It has become bizarrely normal to place your phone by your plate at mealtimes, to interrupt a conversation to take a call and to be so attached to your phone that you think nothing of taking it with you into the lavatory.

When you look at the neuroscience, it's not surprising we've all become so addicted. A smartphone's features and apps are cleverly designed to provide us with constant novelty and reward (a complimentary email, a text from a friend, an interesting snippet of news) and to trigger constant hits of a feel-good brain chemical called dopamine. Once the link between action (picking up your phone) and reward has been established, it doesn't matter how sparse those rewards are. In fact, it is the unpredictability that gets us hooked – like a slot machine.

Yet the problem is that having your phone in sight, or even just the sound of it, has been proven to increase cortisol levels in your blood. Cortisol is your stress hormone, your primary fight or flight trigger. Its release can cause spikes in blood pressure, heart rate and anxiety. This means that, when we're permanently scrolling on social or news feeds, we are putting our body under a lot of physiological stress. And when we're jumping from one thing to another all the time – picking up messages, checking social media, scrolling for that titbit of information we need – we not only add to our stress levels, but we reduce our ability to do other things.

LACK OF CONCENTRATION

Dr Adrian Ward from the University of Texas at Austin is a specialist in understanding consumer behaviour. He has done quite a bit of research into how phone use affects our ability to concentrate, and his studies focus on the extent to which just having your phone around can affect your cognitive capacity.

'We know it's a bad idea to try texting when you're driving, and to scroll through social media when you're studying,' he says. But, on top of that, the 'ping' of a notification or the lighting-up of your screen can make you feel anxious enough to impair performance.

Just having a phone on your desk when you're trying to work can impact your ability to focus.[64]

So what's going on? 'We have a limited amount of cognitive capacity that we use for reading, thinking, talking and being creative,' Dr Ward explains, but because we get such a powerful sense of reward from the various apps on our phone, it is very hard to resist reacting when it pings. 'Even if we're not consciously paying attention to the phone, we will be subconsciously resisting the urge to pick it up – and the process of controlling this background urge can be quite depleting of your cognitive resources,' he says.

Interestingly, his studies show that we are just as distracted when the phone is turned off as when it is turned on – just the sight of your phone provides a constant reminder of all the fun it could offer. 'A modern phone provides so many different attractive, appealing things in one package, it represents, hypothetically, everything that you could be paying attention to that you're not,' says Dr Ward.

THE BENEFITS OF REDUCING PHONE USE

Reducing your phone use – even by a little bit – can have very useful health consequences. In one 2018 study,[65] people were asked to limit their social media use to 30 minutes per day for three weeks – and that was enough for researchers to see significant reductions in loneliness, depression and anxiety.

A study by Swansea University[66] has shown that reducing social media use by just 15 minutes a day can significantly improve our general health and immune function, as well as reducing levels of loneliness and depression. Not all social media is bad: allowing yourself to get sucked into passive scrolling might increase anxiety and stress, but actively posting and interacting with others can boost self-esteem and life satisfaction. The key point is keeping a cap on the amount of time you actually spend on your phone.

Restricting phone use could be good for your posture if it means you spend less time slouched over or craning your neck to read the small print in your hands. In a 2016 study,[67] Korean researchers found that spending four hours or more a day on a smartphone not only led to poor posture but also reduced respiratory function (the ability to breathe well) and eyestrain.

That's because too much doom scrolling can lead to 'text neck' – neck and shoulder pain caused by spending extended periods with your chin dropped towards your chest to look at your mobile phone in your lap. The weight of your head (around 4.5kg) is happily supported by the spine and neck muscles when you are standing or sitting upright, but – according to the laws of physics – tilting the head forwards puts increased loading on the neck and shoulders. At a 45-degree angle, the load on the spine could increase to 22kg, according to a 2014 study by New York Spine Surgery & Rehabilitation Medicine published in the journal *Surgical Technology International*.[68]

You only need to limit your phone use by a small amount to achieve a positive impact. One large study in Sweden,[69] which looked at the behaviours of over 7,000 young adults, found that sending fewer texts was linked to lower levels of neck and upper back pain.

Stopping doom scrolling at bedtime and moving your phone away from the bed could be enough to improve the quality and duration of your sleep, too.[70]

It is probably unrealistic to suggest people give up their phones entirely, since our phones have become so inextricably entwined into modern life. But it is clear that going phone-free, even for short periods throughout the day, can have surprisingly big benefits. In one study,[71] German researchers asked 619 adults to either continue as normal, to not use their phone for a week, or to reduce their daily use by an hour. Compared to the group who kept using their phones as normal, both the 'total abstainers' and 'reducers' felt less anxious and more satisfied with life. But what was really interesting was that three months later it was the 'reducers', not the 'total abstainers', who continued to see the most benefits.

just one thing

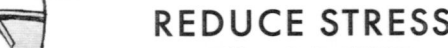

REDUCE STRESS

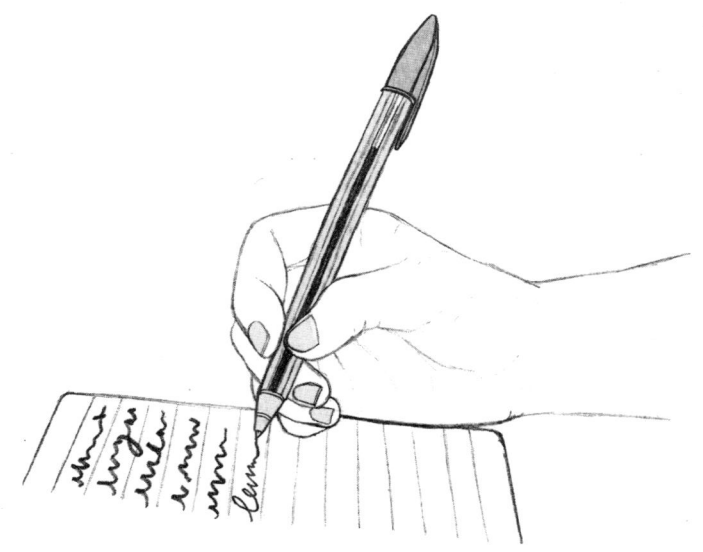

write it down

How to do it: Spend 15 minutes writing about your thoughts and emotions.

Why do it? Journalling is associated with an improvement in mental and physical health, including focus, performance, sleep, immunity and healing.

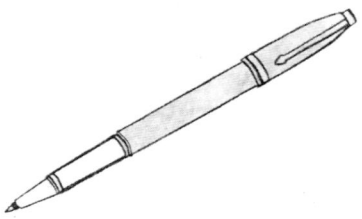

In an age of endless scrolling, perpetual alerts and digital distraction, the simple act of picking up a pen and writing down your thoughts might seem quaint – irrelevant, even. But science suggests it may be one of the simplest and most effective habits you can adopt to boost your health. This is not about journalling for posterity or literary craft. You don't need to be the next Virginia Woolf or Alan Bennett. What matters is the process, not the prose.

This kind of writing, known as expressive writing, involves setting aside 10 or 15 minutes to honestly record your thoughts and emotions – particularly those you might normally avoid or suppress. And the results can be profound. Studies suggest that expressive writing may help you sleep better, think more clearly and even heal faster. It's free, low-effort and entirely private – yet it's backed by decades of psychological and medical research.

HEALTH IMPROVEMENTS

Professor James Pennebaker, a social psychologist at the University of Texas at Austin, has spent nearly four decades studying the link between writing and health. 'The original idea,' he says, 'was to find out whether there were any benefits to disclosing emotions that had been kept secret. What we discovered was rather astonishing.' In his first study,[72] participants were asked to spend 15 minutes on three or four days writing about upsetting experiences. Another group were asked to write about superficial topics. His team then kept track of how often the participants visited their doctor in the following weeks and months. They found the expressive writing group visited their doctor less frequently and reported better mental and physical health.

More recently, scientists have found that expressive writing before a stressful event, such as an exam, can help offload intrusive thoughts and free up what psychologists call working memory to enable better focus and performance. And the benefits aren't limited to mental clarity. In one experiment,[73] New Zealand researchers asked medical students to write about emotional experiences the day before a routine vaccination. Six months later, those students showed stronger immune responses compared to a control group who had not written anything.

Expressive writing, it seems, has the ability to affect our immune system, our hormones, our sleep – and even our physical healing. In one controlled trial,[74] people who wrote about emotional upheavals healed more quickly after a skin biopsy than those who did not. Asthma sufferers have shown reduced symptoms; arthritis patients have experienced less pain and used fewer medications. And in one small study,[75] women recovering from early-stage breast cancer who took part in writing sessions reported fewer headaches and stomach complaints – and attended fewer medical appointments in the months that followed.

All this from jotting down a few private thoughts? 'It's about allowing yourself to make sense of something that might have been floating around your brain in a vague, unresolved way,' explains Professor Pennebaker. 'Once those thoughts are out, you're less likely to ruminate, which means you can sleep better, connect better with others, and in some cases – heal faster.'

STRESS RELIEVER
The paradox is that writing about negative emotions doesn't worsen your mood; instead, it seems to help regulate it. Studies[76] have

shown that people who practise expressive writing feel calmer and more in control, and that the positive effects can ripple out into their social lives. 'We found that, a month later, people were more sociable, laughed more and even reported being better listeners,' Pennebaker says.

If you're feeling anxious or mentally over-revved, expressive writing is worth a try, especially if your thoughts are preventing you from winding down at night. Unlike talking to a friend or therapist, which can sometimes feel daunting, writing privately offers a judgement-free space where you can be completely honest. You don't need to re-read your words, share them or even keep them. In fact, Pennebaker encourages people to throw their writing away afterwards.

'There are no rules,' he says, 'except one: keep writing. Don't edit. Don't correct. Just write continuously for 10 to 15 minutes.' You can even try what he calls 'finger writing', which involves tracing out the words in the air with your finger – astonishingly, this also works.

Expressive writing isn't a cure-all. If you're dealing with severe trauma, depression or persistent anxiety, professional help is essential. But for the rest of us, it's a remarkably accessible tool. If after two or three days, you find you're not getting anything from it, Pennebaker advises simply to stop. It doesn't work for everyone – but when it does, the effects can be surprisingly powerful.

HOW TO START EXPRESSIVE WRITING

★ Find a quiet space where you won't be interrupted.

★ Get a pen or pencil and some paper.

★ Set a timer for 10 or 15 minutes.

★ Write continuously without worrying about grammar or structure.

★ Focus on your deepest thoughts and emotions.

★ Afterwards, keep or discard what you've written – it's up to you.

Studies suggest that expressive writing may help you sleep better, think more clearly and even heal faster. It's free, low-effort and entirely private – yet it's backed by decades of psychological and medical research.

just
one
thing

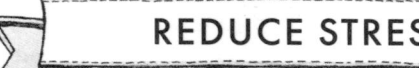

REDUCE STRESS

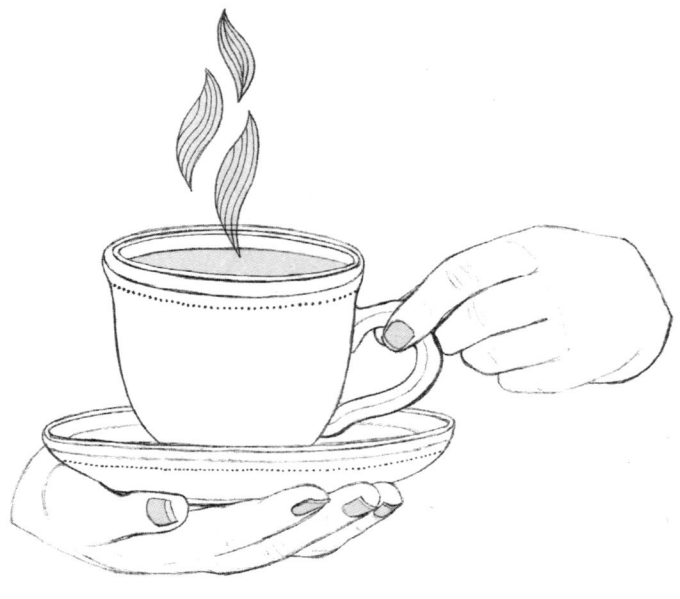

have a cup of tea

How to do it: Drink three cups of black tea (with milk, if you like) a day.

Why do it? It may help to reduce stress levels and enhance mood, memory and bone strength, reducing the risk of heart disease and extending life expectancy.

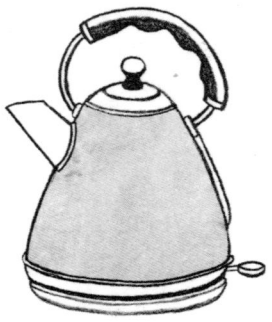

In the UK, we drink millions of cups of tea every single day. It's more than just a beverage – it's a cultural ritual. Whether it's to pause during a hectic work day, mark the end of a long afternoon or sit down with a friend for a chat, the simple act of putting the kettle on offers a sense of comfort and calm.

For many of us, the relaxing effect of tea seems tied more to routine than chemistry: you stop what you're doing, make a warm drink, perhaps have a biscuit, and take a few moments to unwind. But recent scientific research suggests the stress-relieving power of tea may go beyond the psychological. There are, in fact, compounds within the drink itself that can help lower cortisol, boost mood and memory, and even support your heart, bones and longevity.

So if you're not yet a dedicated tea drinker, this might be the perfect moment to pick up the habit.

Our much-loved national drink comes from the leaves of *Camellia sinensis*, an evergreen shrub native to East, South and Southeast Asia. Both green (see page 75) and black tea are made from this plant – the difference lies in how the leaves are processed.

Black tea is fully oxidised, giving it a darker colour and more robust flavour, while green tea is lightly processed to preserve its delicate taste and nutrients.

TIME TO RELAX

One of tea's most important health-boosting compounds is L-theanine, a naturally occurring amino acid that has been shown to promote relaxation without drowsiness. L-theanine increases alpha brainwave activity – a state associated with calm alertness and mental clarity. When paired with the moderate caffeine levels found in tea, this combination seems to improve attention, memory and reaction time, making tea an ideal beverage for staying focused and calm.

In one study,[77] researchers found that individuals who consumed a beverage containing both L-theanine and caffeine felt beneficial effects of sustained attention and memory and were more able to focus. Unlike coffee, which delivers a sharp jolt of caffeine and can lead to jitters or energy crashes, tea offers a gentler lift – enhancing mental clarity while helping you stay cool under pressure.

Professor Andrew Steptoe, a behavioural scientist at University College London, has long studied how lifestyle factors influence stress. He wanted to test whether tea could genuinely reduce stress responses, rather than just provide a comforting ritual. His team conducted a double-blind, placebo-controlled study involving 75 male volunteers.[78] Half were asked to drink four cups of black tea a day for six weeks; the other half consumed a similar-tasting placebo with none of the active compounds.

At the end of the study period, participants were subjected to stress-inducing tasks such as delivering an impromptu speech and solving mental arithmetic under time pressure. Their heart rates, blood pressure, cortisol levels and subjective feelings of stress were all measured.

'We found that both groups showed increased stress responses during the tasks,' says Steptoe. 'But those who drank real tea recovered more quickly afterwards. Their cortisol levels dropped more rapidly, and they reported feeling calmer.'

The researchers believe L-theanine plays a key role. It appears to interact with receptors in the brain associated with GABA (gamma-aminobutyric acid), a neurotransmitter known to promote relaxation and inhibit stress. 'GABA is involved in calming the nervous system,' explains Steptoe. 'By increasing its activity, L-theanine may help reduce anxiety and promote faster recovery from stress.'

GOOD FOR YOUR HEART AND BONES

Tea's benefits don't stop at brain health. Increasing evidence suggests it can also support cardiovascular health and even protect against brittle bones. In one long-term population study,[79] researchers tracked the tea-drinking habits of more than 1,000 women over the age of 75. They found that those who drank three or more cups a day were 30 per cent less likely to suffer a fracture due to osteoporosis than those who drank one cup or fewer per week.

The most likely reason is the fact that tea is rich in plant polyphenols – natural antioxidants that help reduce inflammation and oxidative stress (a chemical imbalance that can lead to cell damage) in the body. These compounds may help slow the rate of bone loss and promote mineral density. Polyphenols also support heart health by improving blood vessel function and reducing the clumping of platelets in the blood.

Steptoe's team also looked at tea's impact on inflammation and platelet activation – two factors that play a major role in heart disease. 'We found that people who drank tea had lower levels of inflammation markers and less platelet activation,' he says. 'This helps us understand why large-scale studies have shown lower rates of heart attacks and strokes among tea drinkers.'

Perhaps the most compelling evidence comes from a major UK study[80] that analysed data from nearly half a million people. The researchers found that those who drank two or more cups of tea a day had a significantly lower risk of dying over an 11-year period than non-tea drinkers – even after adjusting for lifestyle, socio-economic status and other health factors.

Importantly, this protective effect remained regardless of whether people added milk or sugar to their tea, reinforcing the idea that the tea itself – rather than the surrounding ritual – is responsible for the health boost.

HOW DO YOU TAKE YOUR TEA?

Part of tea's appeal lies in its versatility. There are hundreds of blends and varieties, from robust English breakfast to fragrant Earl Grey, and from soothing chamomile to invigorating green tea. You can enjoy it hot or iced, with milk, lemon or honey.

Drinking tea without milk may be helpful; some studies suggest that milk proteins can bind to beneficial polyphenols such as catechins, slightly reducing their antioxidant activity. However, research indicates that the health effects are less dependent on whether you add milk or sugar, and more on how strong you brew it. 'The longer the steeping time, the more of those beneficial bioactive compounds are released,' says Professor Steptoe. Allow your tea to brew for at least 3–5 minutes to extract the maximum amount of polyphenols.

Tea contains more than 200 active compounds, many of which remain only partially understood. As research continues, scientists may yet discover new mechanisms behind its beneficial effects. But for now, the evidence is already impressive. Tea supports mental clarity, helps reduce stress, promotes heart and bone health, and may even contribute to a longer life. And with no downside – provided you don't overdo the sugar or drink excessive amounts – it's one of the easiest health habits to adopt.

So, what are you waiting for? Pop the kettle on, dunk that tea bag, and enjoy the gentle lift and lasting benefits of the UK's favourite brew.

just
one
thing

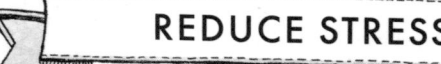

REDUCE STRESS

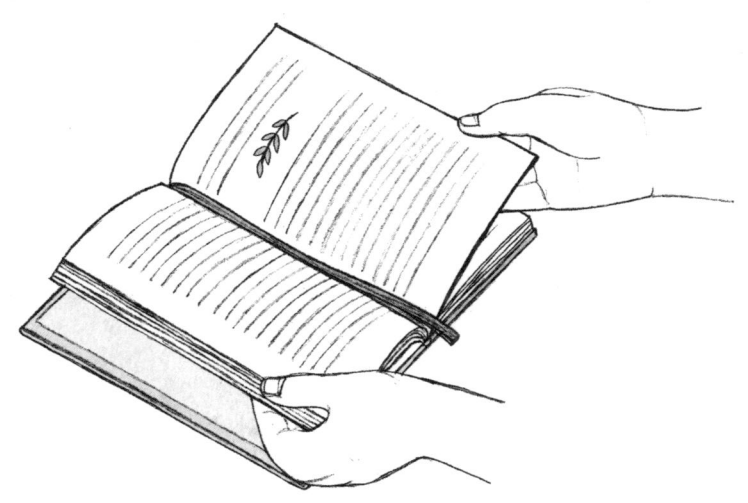

read a poem

How to do it: Spend five minutes a day reading poetry out loud.

Why do it? Reading poetry can ease stress, lift the mood and support heart and immune health.

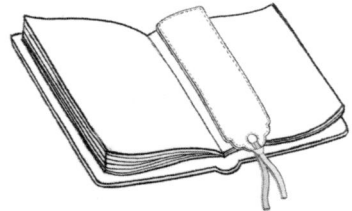

For centuries, poetry has been a way to express love, grief, joy and longing. It is a form of emotional shorthand that distils complex feelings into a few carefully chosen lines. But now, research is beginning to show that verse may do far more than move us emotionally. It turns out that reading poetry has a multitude of mental and physical health benefits.

The idea of healing through verse stretches back to ancient Egypt, where words written on papyrus were dissolved in liquid and drunk as a remedy. But while modern medicine is no longer served in a cup of ink, there is growing evidence that poetry – especially when read aloud – can activate the body's parasympathetic nervous system, the 'rest and digest' response that counterbalances the adrenaline-fuelled stress state of modern life.

In one study involving 44 hospitalised children,[81] those who either read or wrote poetry saw reductions in sadness, anger, worry and fear – and reported increased energy levels. Another trial, of cancer patients in the USA,[82] found that while both music and poetry improved mood and pain levels, only the group of participants who read poetry showed increased feelings of hope.

There's clearly something wonderfully healing in verse, and poetry therapy is now increasingly used in clinical settings – including in schools, prisons, psychiatric wards and hospices – to help people explore their emotions, find comfort or process trauma. While the research remains limited, early findings are encouraging. In a 2022 survey of 400 poetry enthusiasts by researchers at the universities of Plymouth and Nottingham Trent,[83] participants reported that reading, writing and discussing poetry helped them cope with feelings of loneliness, anxiety and depression. Most had already been drawn to poetry before the study, so the findings may be partly self-selecting, but the emotional resonance of verse – particularly when shared – appears to be a common theme.

Many poems – even those that touch on grief or despair – end with a sense of transformation, understanding or beauty. That, coupled with the inherent structure and flow of the lines, can offer both emotional and physiological relief.

Reading poetry forces you to naturally slow down and notice not just the meaning of the words, but the rhythm, imagery and emotional resonance of the verse. Poems can give language to complex emotions such as grief, longing, joy or wonder, allowing readers to acknowledge these states gently. It is almost like a form of guided meditation or mindfulness, as the words prompt reflection and heightened awareness.

IT'S ALL IN THE BREATHING PATTERNS

Quietly listening to or reading poetry is clearly beneficial, but speaking it aloud adds another layer of calm. In a small but intriguing study by researchers at the Swiss Association of Art Therapies,[84] reading rhythmic poetry was shown to regulate breathing patterns, slow the heart rate and increase heart rate variability (HRV) – a measure of the body's capacity to respond to stress. The researchers found that this shift was even *more* pronounced than when participants practised deliberate deep-breathing exercises.

'The key is rhythm,' explains Dietrich Von Bonin, who led the study. 'When you read rhythmic poetry aloud, your breathing naturally slows and lengthens. This stimulates the parasympathetic nervous system, which supports everything from digestion to immune function and mood.'

It has long been known that our breathing patterns are tightly linked to our autonomic nervous system, which has two branches: the sympathetic and the parasympathetic nervous systems. The sympathetic system activates the 'fight or flight' response that speeds up heart rate and increases alertness, and the parasympathetic system is the 'rest and digest' response which slows the heart rate, promoting calm and recovery. The balance between these two systems shifts throughout the day – our heart rate naturally rises slightly when we inhale and falls slightly when we exhale – but breathing is one of the few ways we can influence that balance.

That's why breathing exercises that encourage us to exhale slowly, making the exhale longer than the inhale, can be so deeply relaxing. Slow, prolonged exhalations mechanically signal your brain via stretch receptors in the lungs that 'things are safe', allowing the vagus nerve to ramp up parasympathetic signals. This reduces heart rate, lowers blood pressure and shifts your body chemistry towards calm.

In Von Bonin's study, participants were divided into three groups: one read hexameter verse (a structured, rhythmic poetic form where each line has six main accented syllables), one practised slow breathing (keeping to 12 breaths per minute), and a third group just breathed normally. The researchers fully expected structured breathing exercises which emphasised extending the exhale to work best, but to their surprise, the group reading poetry showed the greatest synchronisation between breath and HRV. This synchronisation – essentially, the breath and heart working in harmony – is considered a sign of a well-regulated nervous system.

The finding suggests that the natural cadence and structure of rhythmic poetry may offer a more intuitive, engaging way to access relaxation – one that doesn't rely on remembering to breathe deeply or hold a certain posture. There's an important physiological component to this. As you read rhythmically, your exhalation tends to lengthen. 'In our studies, those reading the poetry naturally breathed out for three times as long as they breathed in,' Von Bonin explains. 'That's the sweet spot for switching on the relaxation response.'

Not all poetry has this effect, however. For the benefits to kick in, rhythm matters. The poetry must include a regular pattern of stressed and unstressed syllables, ideally with longer lines that allow the breath to flow. Sonnets, blank verse and epic poetry are often good examples. That's why Von Bonin used hexameter poetry, which is often found in classical Greek and Latin poetry and is characterised by a rhythmic combination of stressed and unstressed syllables. Think of the sound of a galloping horse: 'DA-da-da DA-da-da DA-da-da DA-da-da DA-da-da DA-da-da'. This appears to provide a particularly potent rhythm for physiological synchronisation.

Unfortunately, it's not easy to find the right kind of poetry to exact this response. Most of us might be more in tune with Sylvia Plath, Rudyard Kipling, Keats or Yeats than with Homer's *Iliad*. But slightly more modern equivalents may include the work of poets like Henry Wadsworth Longfellow, whose 1847 poem *Evangeline* is written in hexameter.

But what matters most is the beat of the poem you are reading. It needs to have a musicality that shapes your breath without conscious effort. 'It doesn't have to be in hexameter,' Von Bonin clarifies. 'But the poetry needs to have a rhythmic structure. Free verse or very short, irregular lines don't produce the same effect.'

In an ideal world, the rhythm, cadence and structure of the poem can provide a scaffolding for relaxation, while the emotional weight offers comfort, resonance and joy. Von Bonin recommends finding rhythmic poems you like and then reading aloud for 5–10 minutes, three or four times a week. He suggests starting small and choosing poems that feel emotionally resonant. 'If the poem is meaningful to you, you're more likely to stick with it,' he says. 'And the emotional content adds to the effect – it increases satisfaction and helps you engage.'

'Any physical activity that slows you down, engages your breath and uplifts you emotionally is good for your health,' says Von Bonin. 'Poetry does all three.'

POETRY PLEASE

When choosing poetry to read aloud, look for poems with a clear metrical structure (a regular pattern of stressed and unstressed syllables) and lines that are a moderate length (six or more syllables). Avoid very short or erratic structures. Go for verse forms such as iambic pentameter (sometimes used by Shakespeare, with lines of 10 syllables, arranged in an alternating pattern of unstressed and stressed syllables), dactylic hexameter (used by Homer and Longfellow), blank verse (with regular metrical but unrhymed lines) or traditional rhyming stanzas. Here are some examples to try:

* ★ 'Still I Rise' (1978) by Maya Angelou
* ★ 'If We Must Die' (1919) by Claude McKay
* ★ '"Hope" Is The Thing With Feathers' (1891) by Emily Dickinson
* ★ 'The Prelude' (1850) by William Wordsworth
* ★ 'Remember' (1849) by Christina Rossetti
* ★ 'Evangeline' (1847) by Henry Wadsworth Longfellow
* ★ 'To Autumn' (1819) by John Keats
* ★ 'Sonnet 18' ('Shall I compare thee to a summer's day?'; 1590s) by William Shakespeare

Here are some suggestions for finding poetry:

* ★ The Poetry Archive (www.poetryarchive.org) offers free recordings of poets reading their work.
* ★ Poetry Foundation (www.poetryfoundation.org) is a searchable database of thousands of poems.
* ★ Apps such as Poem-a-Day or Poesi are a good resource.
* ★ Anthologies like Staying Alive (edited by Neil Astley, Bloodaxe Books, 2002) or The Nation's Favourite Poems (BBC Books, 1996) offer many excellent choices.

POETRY MINDFULNESS

How to turn poetry reading into a mindfulness exercise:

1. PICK A POEM THAT RESONATES WITH YOU. If you're unsure which poem to pick, just start with something short such as a haiku, a sonnet or a single stanza.

2. FIND A COMFORTABLE, QUIET SPOT. Remove distractions and, if helpful, set a timer for 5–10 minutes.

3. READ THE POEM ALOUD, SLOWLY. Savour each word. Notice how your breath moves with each line. Let the rhythm guide your breath. Repeat lines if they feel good. Remember, you're not studying – you're unwinding.

4. AFTER READING A STANZA OR LINE, PAUSE. Close your eyes and notice the images, emotions or physical sensations that the poem evokes.

5. REFLECT AFTER READING. When you finish reading, take a moment to reflect. What thoughts, feelings or sensations linger?

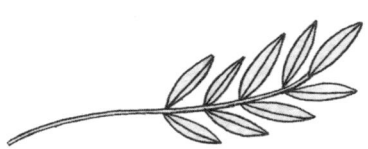

just one thing

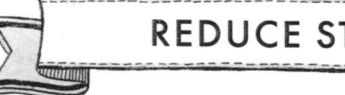

REDUCE STRESS

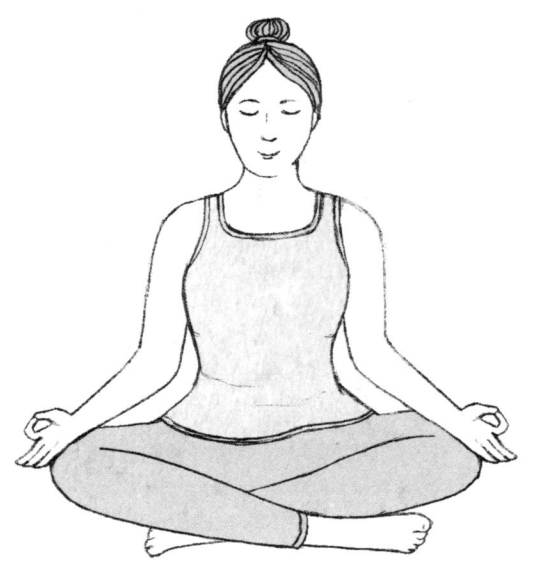

practise yoga

How to do it: Take regular yoga classes.

Why do it? Practising yoga may ease stress and chronic pain; lower blood pressure; boost mood, learning and memory; improve sleep; and slow the ageing process.

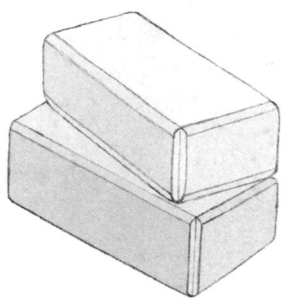

Your yoga journey might begin with a few simple stretches on a mat, but the benefits of yoga go far beyond flexibility. Once seen as a niche pursuit, yoga has become a fast-growing wellness trend – and with good reason. Research shows that regular yoga practice – whether you're doing 10 minutes of gentle breathing from the comfort of an armchair or an hour of flowing movement in a heated studio – offers a powerful way to reduce stress, build resilience and support both physical and mental health at any age. And you don't need to twist yourself into a pretzel or chant mantras to benefit.

Yoga is said to have originated in India over 5,000 years ago. However, it only started to become really popular worldwide towards the end of the 19th century, when developments in photography meant pictures of the poses and exercises started to spread between India and the West.

Now yoga is widely acknowledged as a great way to improve flexibility and balance, increasing strength and improving posture and body awareness. But fascinating studies now show it to be particularly effective at helping to reduce stress and anxiety and to slow the pace of ageing.

There are a wealth of different variants, including vinyasa yoga, Ashtanga yoga, hot yoga and even chair yoga. Yet, if you are particularly interested in testing out yoga's impact on brain health, then the majority of studies have looked at hatha yoga, which combines classic yoga poses with slow, deep breathing.

A German study from 2018[85] compared brain scans of participants before and after 10 weeks of either hatha yoga or playing sport, and found that the yoga group saw significant increases in the grey matter density in the hippocampus, a brain region associated with learning and memory.

Yoga is also well known for its positive effect on mental wellbeing. In a small 2017 pilot study,[86] participants with mild to moderate depression were randomised into groups that either practised yoga or attended a yoga history class for 90 minutes twice a week for eight weeks. By the end of the study, 60 per cent of the yoga group were no longer classified as clinically depressed, compared to only 10 per cent in the history group.

It seems that yoga helps reduce levels of the stress hormone cortisol and regulates our sympathetic nervous system, which controls the body's stress response. These effects, along with lower levels of inflammatory markers, are thought to be the main reasons behind yoga's impact on anxiety and depression.

THE SECRET OF ETERNAL YOUTH?

Exciting new research suggests regular yoga practice could even benefit us at the cellular level by boosting mitochondrial function to slow the pace of ageing. Mitochondria are tiny power units that live inside our cells and provide us with energy. The better they're working, the better we function. But as we get older, these mitochondria can get damaged or develop mutations. When that happens, they become less efficient at producing energy. This gradual energy decline is one of the key reasons our tissues and organs don't work as well as we age.

Professor Rima Dada, from the All India Institute of Medical Sciences in New Delhi, has been studying the benefits of yoga on lifestyle diseases such as diabetes by looking at energy production at the cellular level. Her research[87] has shown that practising yoga may help slow the development of lifestyle diseases because it appears to protect both mitochondrial health and the DNA inside our cells. It does this by switching on certain genes that help repair DNA, reduce harmful stress on cells, and boost the body's natural antioxidant defences (which protect us from damage caused by things like pollution, poor diet and stress).

'Diseases such as diabetes, coronary artery disease, hypertension, depression and cancer have some common underlying mechanisms, such as inflammation and oxidative stress,' she says. 'When we looked at rheumatoid arthritis for instance, which is a very severe, chronic, progressive, inflammatory autoimmune form of arthritis, we found that practising yoga can actually decrease levels of inflammation.'

In her trials,[88] she took two groups of patients who had been given anti-rheumatic drugs and asked one group to practise yoga as well. They practised five days a week, for one hour, for eight weeks. 'At the end of the trial, we measured a decrease in levels of inflammatory cytokines, which indicates a lowering of oxidative stress in the yoga group,' she says. 'Levels of stress and the rate of ageing of immune cells dropped as yoga appeared to help restore the immunological balance.'

Not only did these patients have a measurable decrease in inflammation, but they also recorded lower levels of pain and stiffness, which meant they were better able to perform their day-to-day activities. 'They reported an improvement in the quality of life and also a decrease in the severity of depression,' she adds.

DEEP RELAXATION

So what's going on? Professor Dada explains that good yoga practice is made up of three important parts: physical postures (called asanas), breathing exercises (known as pranayama) and meditation. In combination, these three help to calm your mind – often putting you in a meditative, relaxed state. Levels of cortisol, the body's main stress hormone, start to drop. When cortisol goes down, so does inflammation and oxidative stress, which are both linked to disease and ageing.

As stress hormones decrease, the body increases its production of chemicals that support brain health, and this helps the brain to stay flexible and adaptable – a concept known as neuroplasticity. Yoga also activates the parasympathetic nervous system, which is your body's natural 'rest and repair' mode. This helps with everything from digestion to emotional recovery.

Over time, regular yoga practice helps people feel less stressed and more in control. Practising yoga regularly has even been shown to change the structure of the brain – increasing the amount of both grey matter (linked to memory and decision-making) and white matter (which helps different parts of the brain communicate). This all adds up to greater resilience, better mental health and a stronger ability to cope with life's challenges.

Professor Dada is convinced these benefits extend to healthy people, too. 'Just 30 minutes a day would be enough to reduce the incidence of developing these lifestyle diseases,' she says. 'Find a good yoga instructor and explain to the instructor if you have any ailments so the poses and breathing practices can be specially designed for you. No need to try to hold complicated postures as simple variations work well enough as long as you combine them with breathing exercises and meditation.'

Contrary to popular belief, you don't have to be fit or flexible to try yoga. In fact, the more inflexible you are, the more you stand to benefit! And with so many different types of yoga available, you're sure to find one that suits you. As a bonus, you don't need a lot of equipment: just wear some comfortable clothes and find a mat – and you're ready to flow.

WHAT'S THE RIGHT TYPE OF YOGA FOR YOU?

Whether you're after a sweaty workout, deep relaxation or support for mental health, there's a form of yoga to suit most needs and fitness levels. If you're unsure where to start, try a beginner-level hatha or vinyasa class – many studios offer taster sessions or online options.

- ★ **HATHA YOGA.** A good introduction for beginners, hatha is a slower-paced style that focuses on basic postures and breathing techniques. It builds flexibility and balance while promoting calm and mental clarity.

- ★ **VINYASA YOGA.** Sometimes called 'flow' yoga, vinyasa links movement with breath in a more dynamic sequence. Expect to move continuously from one pose to another, making this class more cardiovascular and physically demanding.

- ★ **ASHTANGA YOGA.** This is a rigorous and structured practice involving a fixed sequence of poses performed in a set order. It's physically challenging and suited to those who prefer routine and discipline.

- ★ **IYENGAR YOGA.** This is a slow, precise form of yoga that uses props such as blocks and straps to help you achieve perfect alignment in each posture. It's ideal for those recovering from injury or seeking a more therapeutic approach.

- ★ **YIN YOGA.** A deeply meditative style that involves holding passive stretches for several minutes at a time, yin targets deep connective tissues and is excellent for stress relief and flexibility.

- ★ **RESTORATIVE YOGA.** Focused entirely on relaxation, this style uses blankets, bolsters and props to fully support the body in restful poses. It helps activate the parasympathetic nervous system and calm the mind.

- ★ **HOT YOGA.** A vigorous style of yoga practised in a heated room (typically around 40°C), this helps to increase flexibility through deeper stretches, aiding both fitness and stress reduction.

- ★ **CHAIR YOGA.** This is a gentle, accessible form of yoga suitable for all ages and abilities, with moves that can be adapted to accommodate mobility limitations, injuries or chronic conditions.

THREE KEY YOGA POSES FOR BEGINNERS

1. TREE POSE
- Stand tall with your feet hip-width apart and arms at your sides.
- Shift your weight onto your left foot.
- Place the sole of your right foot against your left ankle, calf or inner thigh, and then bring your hands together in front of your chest (in prayer position).
- Hold for 5 – 10 breaths, keeping your gaze steady on one spot in front of you. If balance is tricky, lightly touch a wall or chair for support.

Benefits: Improves balance, focus and posture.

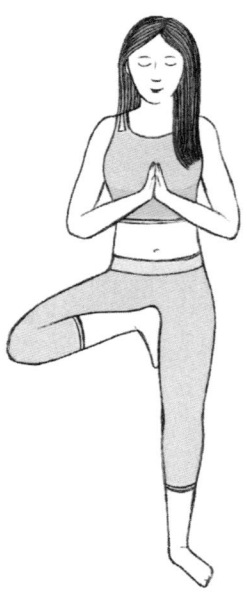

2. DOWNWARD-FACING DOG

- Start on your hands and knees with your wrists under your shoulders and knees under your hips.
- Spread your fingers wide, pressing the palms of your hands firmly into the mat.
- Tuck your toes under and lift your hips towards the ceiling, straightening your legs as much as is comfortable so your body is in an inverted V shape. Keep your head between your arms.
- Press your heels towards the floor and hold for 5–8 breaths.

Benefits: Stretches the back, hamstrings and shoulders, while strengthening the muscles of the arms and core.

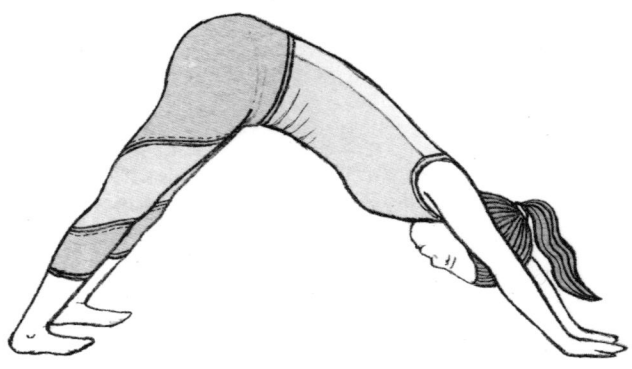

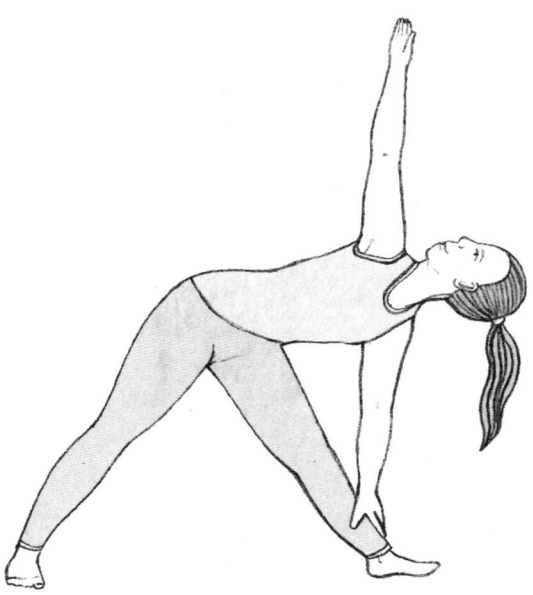

3. TRIANGLE POSE

- Stand with your feet wide apart, and then turn your left foot out 90 degrees and your right foot slightly inwards.
- Extend your arms out to the sides, parallel to the floor.
- Inhale, then exhale as you reach your left arm forwards, tilting your torso over your left leg, keeping the left knee soft. Rest your left hand on your left shin, ankle or a yoga block (wherever you can reach without straining).
- Extend your right arm straight up, opening your chest towards the ceiling, and look up at your right hand.
- Hold for 5–8 breaths, and then switch sides.

Benefits: Stretches legs, hips and spine, while opening the chest and shoulders.

just
one
thing

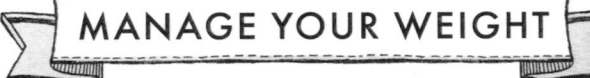

MANAGE YOUR WEIGHT

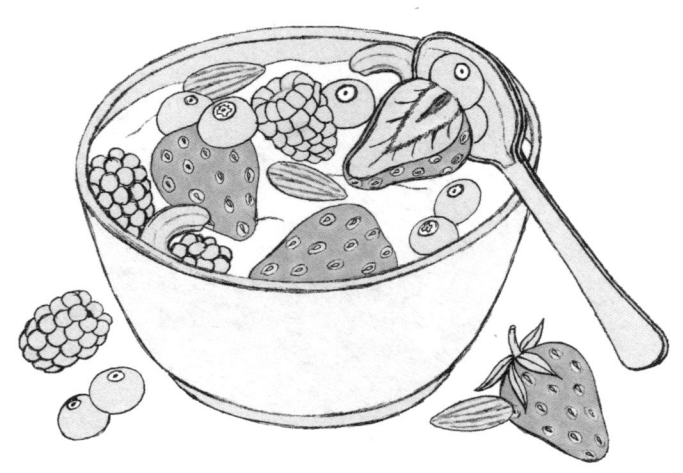

snack smartly

How to do it: Switch some of your unhealthy snacks for healthy ones.

Why do it? Eating healthier snacks may boost mood, steady blood sugar levels, aid weight loss and reduce the risk of heart disease.

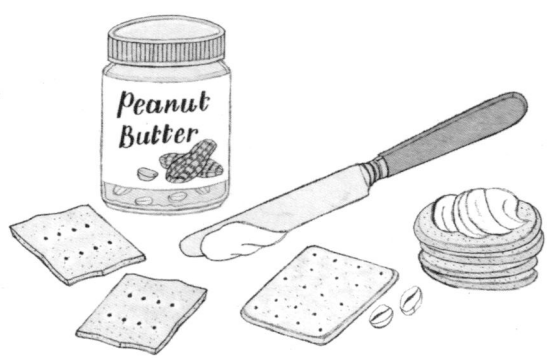

In the quest to improve your diet, it's good to know that changing a few aspects of *how* and *when* you eat a snack can have a big effect on your health. Surveys[89] have shown that, over the last 40 years, we have become a nation of snack-aholics, nibbling, picking and grazing our way through the day.

A snacking habit can seriously increase your calorie load without you realising, but it is also really bad for your health. Unfortunately, three-quarters of the snacks we tend to consume in the UK are heavily processed and high in refined carbohydrates, salt, fat and sugar. Studies[90] have shown that people who regularly snack on processed foods tend to be heavier, and sadly they tend to die younger, too.

But if you've got a sweet tooth or you love the crunch of a crisp, the good news is that you don't have to give up snacks entirely. By simply cutting back on your consumption of processed, starchy, sugary snacks and switching to a few healthier alternatives, you could start to enjoy a multitude of health benefits, including a lower risk of heart disease. Switching out some of your unhealthy snacks could improve your mental health, too. One study of over 400 Brits[91] found that those who ate starchy processed snacks, such as crisps, most days were far more likely to report symptoms of anxiety, stress and depression than those who didn't. By contrast, those who snacked on fruit were less likely to be depressed and more likely to report being in a good mood.

WHEN AND HOW

When it comes to snacking, it's not just what you eat but *when* you eat that's important. Professor Sarah Berry from the Department of Nutritional Sciences at King's College London has been studying the science of snacking. She and her team set out to investigate whether it's the timing of snacks, the quality of snacks or the amount of snacking that does the most damage – and discovered that the biggest issues lie with the quality and the timing, not the quantity.

'We know in the UK that, on average, the snacks that we consume tend to be high in unhealthy nutrients, high in saturated fat, high in refined carbohydrates, high in sugar, and they tend to be low in fibre and healthy proteins,' says Professor Berry. 'It is usually confectionery: biscuits, chocolates, cookies, cakes and crisps. Ninety-five per cent of people confess to snacking, and these "non-meals" are accounting for nearly a quarter of our daily calorie intake,' she says, warning that if you snack on unhealthy foods, the research shows you are much more likely to have higher levels of bad cholesterol and lower levels of good cholesterol. And you're also likely to be carrying more weight around your waist.

However, one of Professor Berry's studies (The Zoe Predict study),[92] which involved 1,000 people, found that snacking on healthy foods – even if you're snacking a lot – is much less likely to increase your health risk. 'Interestingly, we discovered that the time of day matters, too,' she says. The participants in her study who snacked late into the evening ended up with a higher baseline level of blood glucose, poorer insulin sensitivity and alarming levels of blood fat.

'A shocking 30 per cent of people are snacking after nine o'clock in the evening, and even if you're nibbling healthy snacks, late eating of any kind appears to increase your risk of cardiovascular disease,' she says.

The very good news is that switching to healthy snacking can actually have a positive impact on your health. Professor Berry and her team conducted a study[93] to look at the health effects of snacking on nuts. Fifty volunteers were asked to ensure 20 per cent of their energy intake came from almonds each day, and another 50 volunteers had to make sure that 20 per cent of their energy intake was eaten as typical UK snacks. After six weeks, the almond eaters showed a large reduction in LDL cholesterol, the bad type of cholesterol associated with increased risk of heart disease, she reveals. They also had big improvements in a measure of blood vessel function which, according to Professor Berry, translates to a 30 per cent reduction in cardiovascular disease. 'That's a pretty big response when you consider that nothing else in their diet changed,' she adds.

'Snacking is one aspect of our diet that we actually have a lot of control over, so making a few changes is a really great way to improve your health,' says Professor Berry. 'All you need to do is move away from chocolates, crisps and cakes, for example, and to get into the habit of enjoying really healthy snacks that are high in protein, low in sugar, low in refined carbohydrate, and full of healthy oils instead.'

If you're peckish between meals, she recommends making the switch in favour of nuts, fruit, cut-up-vegetables (crudités), a hard-boiled egg or a few spoons of Greek yoghurt or kefir. 'Throw some nuts and some berries into that yoghurt, too!' she suggests. 'People rarely think of cheese as a healthy snack, but as long as you don't eat it in excess, a bit of cheese and a few wholegrain crackers can make a great snack. Food is there to be enjoyed. It's part of our culture, it's part of our social pleasure. And as long as you're not eating ultra-processed crackers all day, every day, and if you're pairing them with cheese, they make a reasonably healthy snack, in my opinion.'

She recommends using the same principles when choosing snacks as we should be using for our main meals: try to avoid heavily processed foods that are high in sugar, higher in refined carbohydrates and low in bio-actives such as polyphenols and fibre. Aim to build a mini healthy meal that has healthy oils and healthy protein that's high in fibre and high in unprocessed ingredients.

HEALTHY SNACKS

★ **ALMONDS, WALNUTS, HAZELNUTS OR PISTACHIOS:** These are a great source of healthy fats, protein, fibre, vitamin E and magnesium.

★ **SEEDS:** These are high in plant-based protein, fibre and minerals like magnesium, zinc and iron. Chia and flaxseeds also deliver omega-3.

★ **SEEDED CRACKERS:** This snack offers slow-release energy and fibre from the wholegrains, plus nutrients from the seeds.

★ **FRUIT:** Contain vitamins, minerals, antioxidants and fibre for immunity. Dates, figs, prunes and apricots are good sources of potassium.

★ **NATURAL OR GREEK YOGHURT WITH BERRIES AND SEEDS:** Yoghurt provides calcium, protein and probiotics for gut health, berries bring antioxidants and polyphenols, and seeds add omega-3 and fibre.

★ **VEGETABLE STICKS WITH HUMMUS:** This combination offers vitamins, fibre, protein, healthy fats and minerals including iron.

★ **HARD-BOILED EGGS:** Each egg contains 6g of protein.

★ **HOMEMADE NUT AND SEED ENERGY BITES:** These contain fats, fibre and protein. You can find plenty of recipes online.

★ **OATCAKES OR WHOLEGRAIN CRACKERS WITH NUT OR SEED BUTTER:** This combination contains fibre, healthy fats and protein.

★ **UNSALTED, AIR-POPPED POPCORN:** Fibre plus polyphenols.

★ **DARK CHOCOLATE:** This offers flavonoids for heart and brain health.

★ **MINI CHEESE PORTIONS:** Contain protein and calcium for bone health.

★ **SMOOTHIES CONTAINING SOME VEGETABLES:** These are a source of vitamins, minerals and antioxidants.

just
one
thing

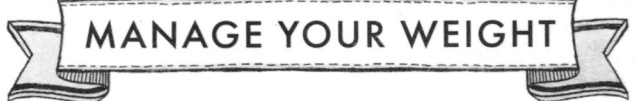

MANAGE YOUR WEIGHT

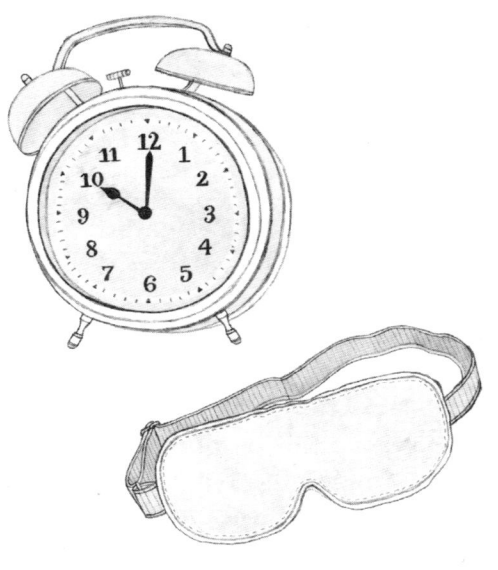

get an early night

How to do it: Go to bed an hour earlier than usual.

Why do it? This can boost mood and reduce the risk of weight gain, depression, heart disease and dementia.

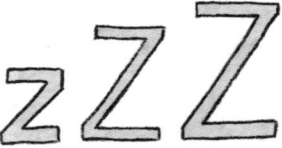

It turns out there's some truth in the old saying: 'Early to bed, early to rise, makes you healthy, wealthy and wise.' Well, the wealthy bit might be stretching things, but emerging research really does show that beginning your bedtime routine an hour earlier than whatever has become your normal can be really beneficial.

If you're a lark who loves to snuggle up in bed and sets an early alarm each morning, you might have been accused of being a tiny bit boring by the owls in your life. But it turns out that the more hours of sleep you can squeeze in before midnight, the better you'll be able to protect your heart, mood and brain.

For starters, getting an early night – that means lights out at around 10 or 11pm – can boost your mood. Studies have shown that people who go to bed earlier have fewer negative thoughts than those who go to bed later. A recent study[94] of over 800,000 people by researchers from Harvard, MIT and the University of Colorado found your risk of depression is linked to the timing of your sleep midpoint (halfway between your bedtime and wake time). Based on this, they conclude that if someone who normally goes to bed at 1am were to go to bed an hour earlier, they could reduce their risk of depression by 23 per cent, theoretically at least. Two hours earlier could reduce it by a whopping 40 per cent.

One suggested explanation is that shifting your bedtime earlier means you've got a better chance of getting extra hours of light in the morning, which should prompt your body to release more feel-good hormones and helps to reset your circadian clock, which has a powerful influence on your mental and physical health. This effect is likely to be more pronounced in the summer months when the days are longer and morning light is more intense, but even in winter, outdoor light exposure still acts as a time cue for your circadian rhythm. Disrupting this rhythm, by staying up late, can increase your risk of metabolic problems and mood disorders, and it can weaken your immunity.

Getting an early night can also benefit your brain in measurable ways, because when you are in deep sleep, your body clears toxins from your brain. This deep, restorative sleep tends to occur in the first part of the night (10pm to 2am), so going to bed a bit early helps you to capture more of this stage, which is crucial for memory consolidation. If you go to bed late, you don't shift this deep sleep forwards, you simply lose some of it.

This was shown in a fascinating study from Boston University[95] where the researchers discovered that, during deep sleep, a wave of cerebrospinal fluid, the liquid that sits around your brain and spinal cord, rushes in and washes away waste that has accumulated during the day. This could help explain why night owls (who typically go to bed late) are more likely to suffer from neurological problems as well as psychological ones.

If that wasn't enough, enjoying an early night could also be very good for your heart health. A study[96] that analysed the sleeping habits of more than 100,000 Brits found that those who went to bed between 10pm and 11pm were 25 per cent less likely to develop heart disease over a five-year period than those who went to sleep at midnight or later.

APPETITE REGULATION

Last but by no means least, shifting your bedtime may also help you regulate your appetite. Professor Esra Tasali from the University of Chicago Sleep Center has conducted in-depth studies into the relationship between sleep and calorie intake.

'We knew from laboratory studies that sleep deprivation increases appetite and increases cravings for higher-carbohydrate food, which means there's a really strong link to weight gain,' says Professor Tasali. 'But we didn't know if we could do anything about it in real life.' She and her team took 80 people who were overweight, and who were habitually sleeping less than six and a half hours a night.[97] Without giving them any dietary or exercise advice, they randomly selected half to continue their habitual sleep habits and asked half to extend their sleep through personalised sleep counselling.

Her team then tracked the participants' energy intake by asking them to drink a modified kind of water that can track energy consumption and expenditure (called 'doubly labelled water', the oxygen and hydrogen molecules are replaced with slightly altered elements that allow calories consumed and burned to be accurately measured through urine or saliva samples). The results showed that the group which extended their sleep by going to bed just over one hour earlier per night consumed 270 kilocalories a day *less* than they had been previously eating. 'This is really huge in terms of weight regulation,' says Tasali. 'If those healthy sleep habits were to be maintained, it would lead to clinically significant weight loss.'

The participants also reported that the early night helped them to function at their best, and they felt more energetic, more alert and happier. The only downsides? Many said they were frustrated that they couldn't watch TV or use the internet as much as they'd like.

Professor Tasali believes this calorie drop happens because good sleep helps us regulate our bodily systems better. 'If we don't quite sleep enough, levels of the appetite-stimulating hormone ghrelin are increased, which makes us feel hungry and tells our brain to eat more,' she explains.

If you're keen to try to go to bed earlier, she believes one of the important things is to find and establish your own individual bedtime routine. 'Get into the habit of doing something that relaxes you at night,' she says. 'That could be reading a book or listening to music, as long as it is conducive to sleep.' She recommends limiting light exposure and staying away from stimulating activities such as scrolling on your phone, catching up on social media or finishing off work-related emails.

It is worth pointing out that this advice doesn't really work for insomniacs who might spend hours and hours in bed at night, fretting over their infuriating wakefulness. But if you're one of many who puts off bedtime because you're watching box sets or scrolling through social media, then this is a top tip for you!

WIND-DOWN ROUTINE

Help your body and brain adjust to your new, earlier bedtime by adopting a calming wind-down routine:

1. THREE HOURS BEFORE BED. Stop eating and start winding down. Aim to finish dinner at least three hours before bed, to allow your body temperature to fall naturally. Late meals can raise core temperature and disrupt melatonin secretion, impeding deep restorative sleep.

2. TWO HOURS BEFORE BED. Adopt a sleep-friendly ambience by dimming lighting and avoiding bright screens. Although the blue-light narrative is overplayed, devices can keep the mind stimulated.

3. ONE HOUR BEFORE BED. Having a warm bath around an hour before bedtime helps trigger changes in the brain which induce sleep. The bath raises your body temperature, increasing the circulation of blood to your skin, hands and feet. When you get out of the bath, your body will continue to radiate heat, but your core temperature will slowly drop over the course of an hour. This signals to your brain that it's time to sleep, supporting deep sleep onset. For the best results, add a few drops of lavender essential oil (vanilla, rose and bergamot oils can also be effective) to the warm water. Soak yourself for at least 10 minutes.

4. BEDTIME. A bedtime ritual – reading a physical book or listening to calm music – actively encourages your brain to slow down. Studies show that slow, calm classical, jazz or folk music (ideally with a rhythm of 60–80 beats per minute) could help you fall asleep faster, sleep longer and wake up less during the night.

just one thing

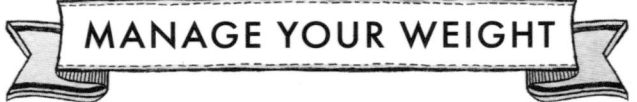

MANAGE YOUR WEIGHT

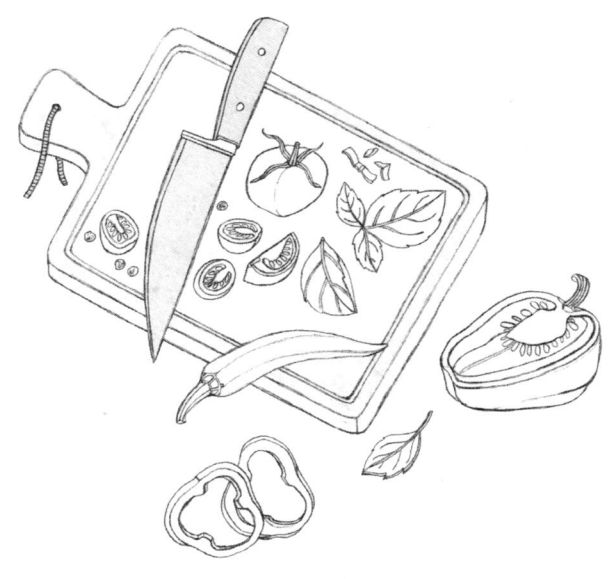

cook from scratch

How to do it: Cook from scratch at least three evenings a week.

Why do it? Home-cooking could reduce calorfic intake and boost nutritional intake, while raising self-esteem.

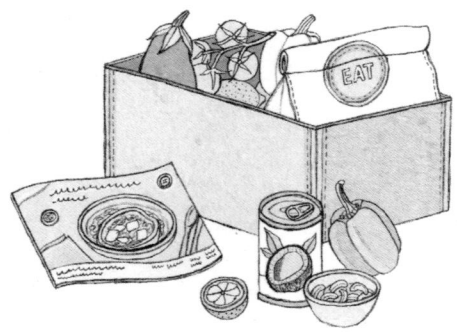

When you're thinking about your evening meal, it is perfectly understandable to be tempted by a takeaway, a ready meal, or something pre-packaged from the supermarket, especially if you're busy and time is tight. But if you want to improve your health and that of your family, it really is best to get back to basics with food, whenever possible. Cooking from scratch doesn't have to be difficult or time-consuming, but eating home-cooked meals could reduce the amount of calories you consume and improve your physical and mental health.

Cooking from scratch means making real food with real ingredients, whether fresh, frozen or dried. Sounds perfectly normal, right? But these days, although we watch a lot of programmes about cooking, we're actually cooking from scratch less than ever before.

A UK YouGov report[98] found that only 23 per cent of Brits cook from scratch most days, 10 per cent do it once a week, and 10 per cent confess they hardly ever cook from scratch at all. Instead, we rely far too heavily on ready meals and takeaways.

ULTRA-PROCESSED FOODS

In the UK, roughly two-thirds of our calories now come from ultra-processed foods (UPFs). These are foods that are typically made in factories and have five or more ingredients, including nasties like emulsifiers and sweeteners that you don't normally use in home cooking. UPFs can be a quick and easy option, but they are often an unhealthy one.

A recent umbrella review published in the *British Medical Journal* involving nearly 10 million people[99] found a clear link between a diet high in ultra-processed foods and 32 harmful health effects, including high risks of heart disease, cancer, type 2 diabetes, poor mental health and early death.

The good news is that cooking from scratch more frequently can have a big positive impact, particularly on your waistline. A study of over 11,000 people[100] found that those who ate home-cooked meals more than five times a week were 28 per cent less likely to be overweight than those who cooked from scratch three times a week or less. Not only were their meals healthier, but researchers say home-cooking also improved their eating behaviour. They snacked less, had smaller portions and more shared mealtimes.

And getting creative in the kitchen could also boost your mental health. Studies in both healthy volunteers and cancer patients have found that learning to cook has a big impact on wellbeing. This could be because when you are cooking from scratch you tend to make healthier food choices, but simply learning a new skill will boost confidence which in turn elevates self-esteem.

Dr Emily Leeming is a nutrition scientist at King's College London. She says whatever you cook from scratch is always likely to be healthier for you than eating something from a packet. Studies show we tend to eat more fruits and vegetables when we cook food from scratch – at least one extra portion per day – which can add up significantly for your health over time.

She points out that the key thing to remember about UPFs is that they're engineered to taste delicious: 'We know that the ingredients that make foods taste good are sugar and fat. Those aren't necessarily bad in themselves, but their presence in foods does tend to mean it's much easier for us to go over our energy needs. And that's when it becomes a problem.'

In one landmark study,[101] researchers invited 20 people into a laboratory for four weeks. Half were allocated ultra-processed foods and the other half were given a minimally processed diet of wholegrains, fruits and vegetables, beans and legumes. All were told they could eat as much or as little as they liked. The study revealed that the people eating UPFs consumed 500 calories more each day than the people on the minimally processed diet. The UPF group gained 1kg in weight and the non-UPF group lost 1kg.

'This study wasn't able to show why this was happening,' says Dr Leeming, 'but subsequent studies[102] have highlighted the fact that we tend to eat processed food too quickly for the signal to get back to our brains to say that we feel full.'

She warns that eating too many UPFs displaces the sorts of foods that our gut bacteria really enjoy – those rich in fibre. 'Without enough plant roughage from fruit and vegetables, wholegrains, beans and legumes, our gut bacteria will struggle to perform all the useful and beneficial functions they normally do for us,' she adds.

In addition, when you cook from scratch, you tend to use less fat, salt, sugar and, of course, artificial additives than if you grabbed a takeaway or defrosted a frozen ready meal. For instance, people who eat a UPF diet tend to eat double the daily recommended amount of salt, which is 6g for adults. 'Salt consumption is linked to elevated blood pressure, which is a risk factor for heart disease,' says Dr Leeming. 'And 70 per cent of the salt we eat doesn't come from sprinkling salt on food – it is hidden in processed foods.'

It's not just our body that benefits. There have been multiple observational trials looking at how cooking from scratch can bring mental health benefits. 'When we are working with our hands, there's good evidence to show it feeds back to the brain and boosts a feeling of satisfaction and contentment,' says Dr Leeming. 'Actually, cooking is sometimes used as a form of therapy because it helps people gain confidence and new skills.'

She suggests that anyone who isn't used to cooking from scratch should start small. 'Find a simple recipe that works for you. It might only use four ingredients, but if you cook that once a week you will be making a significant change,' she says. It's also a good idea to capitalise on the convenience of tinned and frozen foods. One of her biggest tips is to make sure the freezer is well stocked with ingredients: 'Frozen vegetables are packed with nutrients, many of which are retained if you microwave them – it is one of the best ways to cook vegetables,' she says.

'We are always going to need some element of convenience, because who has the time to cook from scratch all day every day?' she adds. 'But once you try cooking a meal, the easier it will become, and every small change you can make creates a much bigger impact long-term.'

Not everyone has access to a kitchen or the resources to cook from scratch. But if you can, then doing so really should have an impressive impact on your waistline, mood and gut microbiome. You don't have to cook anything fancy, you don't need to spend a lot of time on it – it could be pasta in a tomato sauce – but every time you avoid convenience food with a long list of ingredients, you will be benefitting your health.

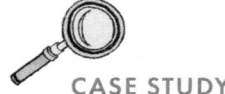

CASE STUDY
Richard, an NHS worker from Belfast
'The only home-cooked meal in my house is a Sunday roast, and pretty much every other meal is convenience foods like takeaways and fast food. So I'm ashamed to say I don't really eat a lot of vegetables. Normally, I don't have the time to prepare meals, but it wasn't too hard once I put my mind to it, and within a couple of days I noticed my digestion starting to improve, I'm sleeping better and my mood is lifted.'

TIPS FOR COOKING MORE OFTEN

1. START WITH JUST ONE MEAL. If you're new to home-cooking, begin by preparing just one homemade meal a week. Choose something simple, like a vegetable stir-fry or a pasta dish with fresh ingredients. As you gain confidence, build up to cooking more frequently.

2. STOCK A BASIC PANTRY. Keep a few essentials on hand so you're always ready to cook. Start with olive oil, garlic, tinned tomatoes, herbs, spices, grains (like rice or pasta) and eggs. This cuts down on shopping trips and means you can whip up a meal more easily.

3. USE SHORT INGREDIENT LISTS. Look for recipes with five or fewer ingredients. Fewer components mean less prep, less stress and fewer chances to go wrong.

4. TRY HOME-DELIVERED MEAL KITS. Although they can be pricey, meal kits are a great way to introduce new recipes and unfamiliar ingredients. A home-delivered recipe box will often contain individual portions of a few exotic ingredients, so you can try them without having to fill your kitchen cupboards with a full range of oils and vinegars. There's no need to squander lots of money on a long-term subscription – just try a trial period, then stock up on the ingredients and make the ones you enjoy a regular part of your cook-from-scratch repertoire.

5. FOLLOW INSPIRING COOKS ON SOCIAL MEDIA. Search for beginner-friendly recipe creators on Instagram, TikTok or YouTube. Many offer quick, visual guides and tips that make new techniques less intimidating. Seeing someone else do it can help demystify the process. If you aren't on social media, borrow an e-cookbook from friends, go to the library or try a recipe from a magazine.

6. BATCH COOK. Make double quantities when you cook and then freeze half so that, when you need a quick meal, you have a healthy, UPF-free option to hand.

7. BUILD SKILLS. Over time, build your cookery skills gradually. Early skills might include chopping an onion properly, making a tomato sauce or roasting vegetables. Small wins add up fast.

BUILD A SHORT CUTS PANTRY

Put together a pantry of pre-prepared ingredients which allow you to cook from scratch with minimal prep time. This is how many professional chefs cook at speed – they call it 'mise en place':

★ Check out the freezer section of your supermarket for chopped onions, mushrooms, peppers and herbs, which can be quickly cooked from frozen. You can buy frozen spinach pellets to throw into curries, pasta and soups, frozen butternut squash cubes for roasting, even frozen avocado chunks for making guacamole or avo toast, as well as the more familiar peas and sweetcorn.

★ Stock up on frozen berries, mango and pineapple chunks to enjoy with yoghurt or for blitzing into smoothies.

★ Search the supermarket shelves for tubes or jars of chopped fresh garlic, chilli and ginger, which save you the fiddle of peeling, grating or mincing.

★ Have a few pouches of pre-cooked rice, lentils, quinoa and couscous ready to use as the base for quick meals.

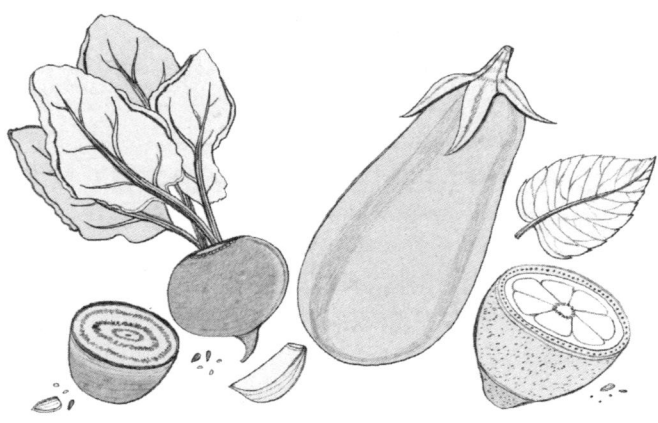

just
one
thing

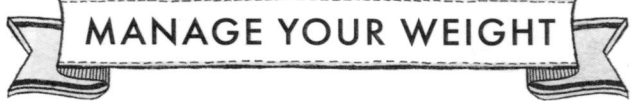

MANAGE YOUR WEIGHT

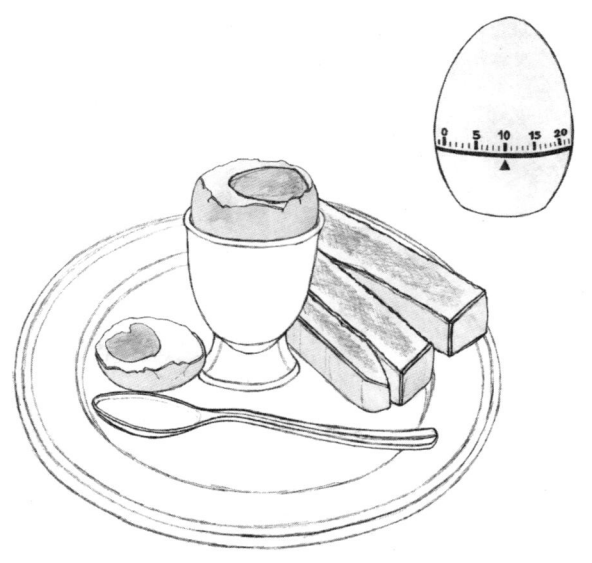

eat slowly

How to do it: Take at least 20 minutes to eat a meal.

Why do it? Slower eating may help with weight maintenance and keeping blood sugar stable, as well as reducing the risk of type 2 diabetes, high cholesterol and high blood pressure.

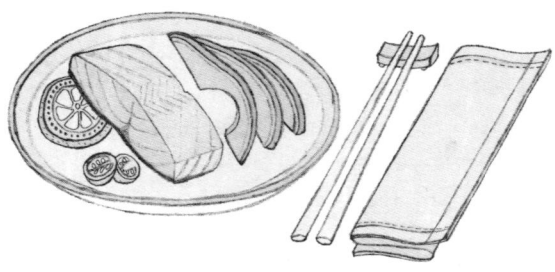

In the UK, we are a nation of speed eaters. On average, we spend just nine minutes eating our evening meal. That's less than half the time we'd typically spend on dinner 50 years ago. Naturally, the speed you eat any meal will be affected by a lot of factors – it can be influenced by what and where you're eating, as well as how you've been brought up. But there's a lot to be said for slowing things down and taking your time.

The human trials in this field are small, but there are some promising findings. It is important to note that slowing down can certainly help you feel fuller for longer. One small study[103] gave identical meals to a group of volunteers. Half the group had to wolf their food down in 6 minutes, while the others were told to take a far more leisurely 24 minutes. Those who ate slowly reported feeling fuller. And three hours later, when both groups were given access to snacks, the people who had eaten slowly consumed 25 per cent fewer calories from the snacks. Blood samples also revealed the speed eaters ended up with higher levels of ghrelin, the hunger hormone, in their system.

Slowing down can improve your blood sugar levels too, which can help reduce your risk of type 2 diabetes. In another study,[104] Japanese researchers asked a group of healthy young women to eat a meal either slowly or quickly, and the next day they ate the same meal at the opposite speed. When the women took just 10 minutes to gulp down the meal, their blood sugars rose faster and stayed higher than when they took 20 minutes to eat exactly the same meal. If your blood sugar is consistently high, it can increase inflammation and your risk of type 2 diabetes.

RISK OF WEIGHT GAIN

There is evidence that, if you eat fast, you are more likely to put on weight and to suffer from metabolic problems such as type 2 diabetes. Observational studies show fast eaters tend to be more overweight, tend to suffer from cardiometabolic diseases like type 2 diabetes, and tend to have high blood pressure and higher blood cholesterol.[105] This finding is backed up by data from longitudinal studies which follow people over a number of years.

But more recently, randomised controlled trials have replicated these findings. In these trials, people are given very specific instructions to either slow down or speed up their rate of eating. One study[106] asked a group of women to slow down the rate at which they were eating – they were given smaller spoons and were asked to chew their food more frequently, and to pause between bites. This meant they extended their eating duration from 10 to 30 minutes, slowing the pace at which the food was being absorbed, and resulting in 65 fewer calories being consumed at each meal.

Professor Sarah Berry from the Department of Nutritional Sciences at King's College London ran a big study looking at the effects of our eating pace on our health. 'We know from observational studies that people who eat their food more quickly have higher levels of obesity and higher levels of cardiometabolic disorders – elevated cholesterol and insulin sensitivity,' she says. 'But there's no clearly defined measurement for what constitutes a fast eater versus a slow eater, so in our studies we typically ask people, compared to an average person, do you think you eat more slowly or more rapidly?'

Around one-third of people confess to being quick eaters, and they tend to be overweight compared to people who eat at a slower or an average pace. 'We also found that faster eaters have a higher energy intake,' she says, revealing that they eat on average 120 extra calories per day compared to the slow or average eaters.

SO WHAT'S GOING ON?

'There are lots of receptors in your lower gut that release particular chemicals that go to your brain,' Professor Berry explains. 'And if you're eating really, really fast, there's no time for the food to reach the receptors, or for the receptors to release the chemicals and for your brain to say, whoa, I've had enough, stop eating!'

Fast eating also results in bigger spikes in blood glucose because your body doesn't have time to release much saliva. 'When you eat slowly, you release more saliva, which stimulates a more effective insulin release, and this reduces circulating blood glucose by removing it from your bloodstream,' she adds.

'The evidence is quite clear that if you're getting through a meal in under 10 minutes you're eating it too fast,' says Professor Berry. 'Ten minutes just isn't enough time for your body to release the gut hormones that control your hunger signalling.'

Her advice is to try to extend most of your meals to last 20 or 30 minutes for maximum benefit to your health.

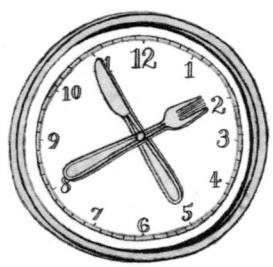

HOW TO SLOW YOUR EATING

Many of us eat on autopilot – grabbing lunch on the go, multitasking during meals or clearing our plate in minutes. But eating more slowly can help you tune into your body's natural hunger and fullness signals, improve digestion and even support weight management. Here are tried-and-tested ways to slow things down:

1. PUT YOUR FORK DOWN BETWEEN BITES. It's a simple trick, but it works. After each mouthful, place your fork or spoon down on the plate. Take a breath, chew fully and only pick up your utensil again when you've swallowed. This small pause helps you reset your pace.

2. USE YOUR NON-DOMINANT HAND. This slows you down and encourages mindful eating.

3. CHEW MORE. Aim to chew each bite around 20–30 times. It sounds like a lot, but it helps break food down properly, aids digestion and gives your brain time to register fullness.

4. DRINK WATER. Having a sip of water between each mouthful is another natural way to slow things down – and we know that having plenty of fluid is great for our health.

5. TRY CHOPSTICKS OR SMALLER UTENSILS. Swapping your usual cutlery for chopsticks or a teaspoon makes you take smaller bites and eat more slowly. It turns a rushed meal into a more deliberate, calm experience.

6. PLAY SLOW, RELAXING MUSIC. Studies[107] show that people who eat while listening to slow music are more relaxed, spend more time eating and chew more times and for longer than those who listen to upbeat music.

7. AVOID DISTRACTIONS. Try not to eat in front of the TV, your phone or a laptop. Focusing on your food helps you better enjoy the flavours – and makes it easier to notice when you've had enough.

8. SET A TIMER OR USE MINDFUL EATING APPS. Apps like *Eat Slower* or *Breathe* can guide your pace with subtle cues. Even setting a timer to stretch your mealtime over 20–30 minutes can help you break the habit of speed eating.

just
one
thing

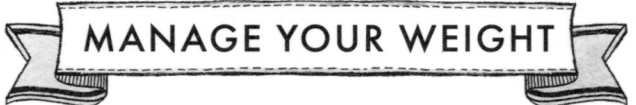

MANAGE YOUR WEIGHT

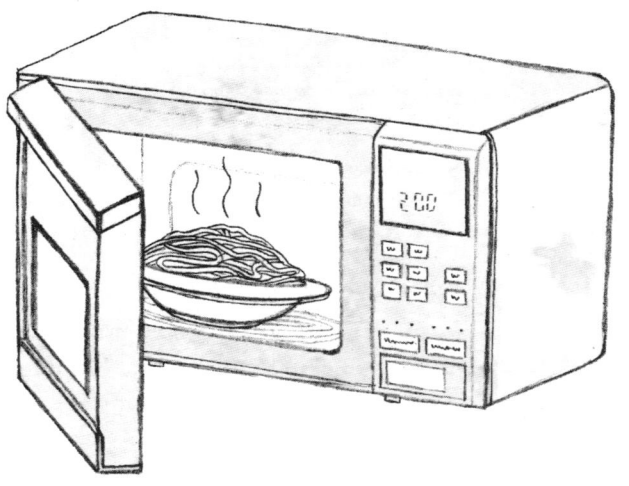

reheat pasta

How to do it: Cook, cool and reheat your pasta, rice and potatoes.

Why do it? It may reduce levels of systemic inflammation and lower the risk of obesity, heart disease, autoimmune disorders and bowel cancer.

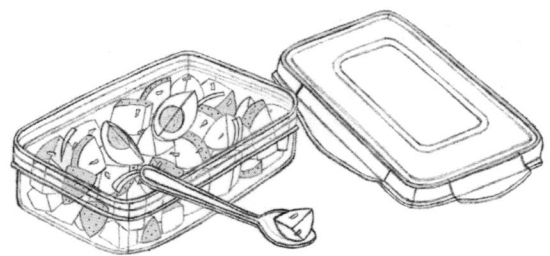

If you've got a tub of last night's pasta sitting in your fridge, don't throw it out! By reheating it, you can transform that humble bowl of penne into a fantastic source of nutrients for your gut bacteria. The process of cooling and reheating a carbohydrate increases its resistant starch – this is a unique type of carbohydrate that, as its name suggests, resists digestion.

Instead of being rapidly broken down into glucose – which spikes blood sugar levels – the starch travels to the large intestine, where it feeds our 'good' gut bacteria and is fermented into substances like butyrate, a short-chain fatty acid that has potent anti-inflammatory effects.

This small change – cooking, cooling and reheating carbohydrates such as pasta, potatoes or rice – transforms how your body handles them. What was once a fast sugar-hit becomes, effectively, a fibrous prebiotic that's gentler on your blood sugar and better for your gut.

'In many ways, resistant starch behaves like fibre,' says Dr Darrell Cockburn, a microbiome researcher at Pennsylvania State University. 'Unlike insoluble fibre, which sweeps the digestive tract, resistant starch ferments slowly, feeding beneficial bacteria and modulating metabolism more subtly. It isn't digested in the small intestine. Instead, it ferments in the colon, producing beneficial compounds like butyrate, which helps keep the gut lining healthy and inflammation in check.'

Cockburn and his colleagues ran a small trial[108] in which volunteers were asked to replace their refined grains with one potato-based dish per day – mashed potatoes, roast potatoes or potato salad. Each potato-based side dish added about 2g of extra resistant starch to their daily diet. 'Potatoes are naturally high in resistant starch and, when you cook them, a lot of the resistant starch remains,' he says, 'but for the study, the dishes were stored frozen and then reheated, in a process which can enhance the resistant starch content.'

Any starchy food can have its resistant starch boosted by going through that cooling or even freezing process. Any type of extended storage at cooler temperatures will enhance the formation of resistant starch by up to 50 per cent, he says.

FEED YOUR MICROBIOME

The resistant starch makes it through to the colon and essentially gets fermented by the bacteria there, encouraging them to produce several different compounds. 'The one we're most interested in is a short-chain fatty acid called butyrate,' says Dr Cockburn. His study showed eating more resistant starch actually increased the number of butyrate-producing bacteria in the gut.

This is important because butyrate is the preferred fuel source for colon cells. It helps maintain the integrity of the gut wall, reducing 'leakiness' – where inflammatory compounds escape into the bloodstream. By bolstering the strength of the gut wall, butyrate helps to reduce chronic inflammation (see page 184), which is associated with everything from heart disease to autoimmune disorders, obesity and bowel cancer.

One landmark study, conducted by researchers at the universities of Newcastle and Leeds,[109] examined nearly 1,000 people with Lynch syndrome, a hereditary condition that increases the risk of certain cancers. Half the participants were given 30g of resistant starch daily for an average of two years; the other half received a placebo. They were tracked for over a decade.

The results? Those on resistant starch were nearly 50 per cent less likely to develop cancers of the upper gastrointestinal tract, including the oesophagus and pancreas. 'These are particularly lethal cancers that are often diagnosed late,' the authors noted. 'That such a simple dietary intervention could have such an effect is extraordinary.'

There's also compelling evidence that resistant starch can help regulate blood sugar levels. One small study[110] found that people at risk of type 2 diabetes who consumed more resistant starch saw improved insulin sensitivity and reduced levels of LDL (low-density lipoprotein, aka 'bad') cholesterol. They even lost more visceral fat than a control group.

Animal studies have hinted at broader benefits. In research on mice[111] that had been infected with a serious autoimmune condition called lupus, those fed resistant starch had healthier gut bacteria, higher butyrate levels and lower markers of inflammation.

COOKING AND COOLING

Resistant starch is found naturally in foods like lentils, beans, wholegrains and green bananas, but it can also be increased in common carbohydrates through a simple bit of culinary trickery. 'Cook your starch – whether it's pasta, potatoes or rice – then cool it overnight,' suggests Cockburn. 'This allows the starch molecules to crystallise into a more resistant form. Reheating them doesn't destroy this effect; in fact, it may enhance it.'

Cooked pasta, for instance, provides 1.2g of resistant starch per 100g, but when you cool and reheat it, those levels rise to 3.5g. The resistant starch in rice rises from 0.5g per 100g when cooked to 2g when cooled and then reheated, and the starch in potatoes trebles from 1g to 3g.

Simply refrigerating and freezing food enhances the resistant starch, too. If you slice a loaf of bread and freeze it, then toast from frozen, you maximise its potential resistant starch content. A slice of wholemeal bread might have 1g of resistant starch, but when you toast that slice from frozen the resistant starch rises to 1.5g. So batch-cooking and refrigerating your carbs is a remarkably easy, inexpensive way to make everyday foods better for you. Best of all, these changes require very little effort. Leftover risotto? Better the second time around. Cold potato salad? A gut-friendly summer staple. Beans and lentils? Already rich in resistant starch – and even more so after a stint in the fridge.

EASY WAYS TO BOOST RESISTANT STARCH IN YOUR DIET

1. COOK ONCE, EAT TWICE (OR THREE TIMES). Prepare larger batches of starchy foods like pasta, rice or potatoes and store them in the fridge. Eat cold as part of a salad or gently reheat for a healthier second (or third) meal.

2. EMBRACE THE POTATO SALAD. Cold cooked potatoes are one of the richest sources of resistant starch. Add olive oil, mustard, a little vinegar and herbs for a gut-friendly side dish. An added bonus is that vinegar may also help reduce post-meal blood sugar spikes.

3. FREEZE AND TOAST YOUR BREAD. Slice wholemeal bread before freezing, and then pop frozen slices straight into the toaster. This not only extends the bread's shelf life but slightly increases the resistant starch content – and reduces food waste.

4. MIX IN MORE LEGUMES. Lentils, chickpeas and beans are naturally high in resistant starch. Stir them into soups, salads or stews. Canned versions are convenient and require no extra prep – just rinse and go.

5. GO (GREEN) BANANAS. Slightly underripe bananas contain a significant amount of resistant starch. There's 4.7g per 100g in an underripe banana, 1.3g in a ripe one (yellow with a few spots) and 0.5g in a very ripe one (brown spotted). That's because, as bananas ripen, enzymes break down the resistant starch into sugars. Slice a slightly underripe banana into yoghurt or porridge for a fibre-rich breakfast that supports your microbiome.

just
one
thing

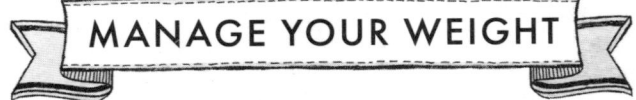

MANAGE YOUR WEIGHT

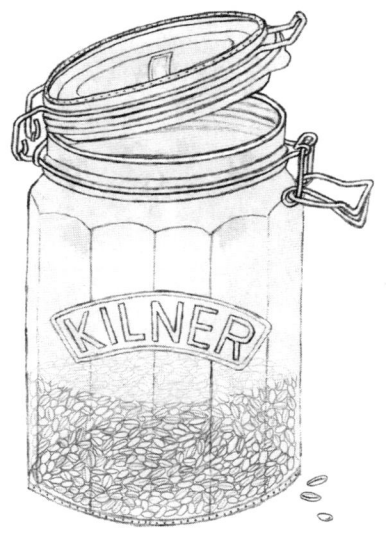

choose
wholegrains

How to do it: Eat three servings of wholegrains (such as brown rice, pasta and bread) a day.

Why do it? It may aid weight loss, lower blood pressure, improve blood sugar levels and reduce cholesterol.

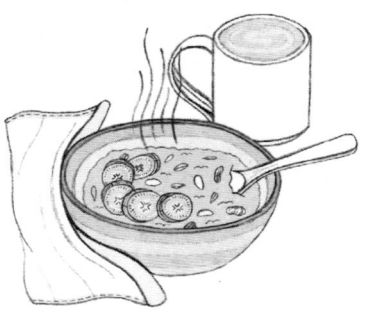

In recent years, carbohydrates – especially grains – have attracted a bad reputation. Many weight-loss diets strictly restrict them. Yet for most of us, there's no need to ditch grains entirely. On the contrary, swapping refined starches for wholegrain alternatives can deliver substantial health gains. Just one 50g portion a day – equivalent to a bowl of porridge or a slice of rye bread – could be enough to slash your risk of getting type 2 diabetes by one-third.

The term 'wholegrains' encompasses a variety of grains, including whole-wheat pasta, wholemeal bread, rolled oats and brown rice. They contain more fibre than the refined grains, such as white rice, bread and pasta, that most of us eat. This fibre boost alone has been shown to help trim your waistline. A meta-analysis of 15 studies with 120,000 participants[112] found people who ate three servings of wholegrains per day were more likely to have a lower body mass index. That's probably because the fibre in wholegrains makes you feel fuller by slowing digestion and influencing the release of gut hormones that tell you to stop eating.

Wholegrains are made up of three parts: the germ or core of the grain, the bran or outer shell, and the starchy endosperm. Refined grains usually have the germ and bran removed. This is a big shame because these are the bits that are packed with healthy fibre, antioxidants, polyphenols, protein and healthy fats. It is these components that contribute to the way wholegrains in the diet can help to lower your blood pressure, improve your blood sugar levels and reduce your cholesterol. Eating them regularly could even help you live longer.

Studies[113] show that switching from a refined to a wholegrain diet can lead to a drop in belly fat and key markers for inflammation (an immune response, often initially triggered by infection, injury or irritation) in just 12 weeks. This is likely to be because losing abdominal fat reduces the number of inflammatory compounds released by the body.

The cardiovascular benefits are also compelling. Harvard researcher Dr Caleigh Sawicki and her team analysed data from more than 3,000 participants who were followed and monitored for over 18 years.[114] She noticed that those with the highest wholegrain intake experienced smaller increases in waist circumference, blood pressure and fasting blood sugar compared to those with the lowest intake.

Sawicki is clear that wholegrains differ significantly from refined grains in both nutritional profile and, importantly, in physiological effect. 'Wholegrains are higher in fibre, important nutrients, antioxidants and polyphenols that are removed during the refining process,' she explains. 'Fibre's primary benefit is the way it absorbs water, expanding in your stomach and moving slowly through your digestive system. This can make us feel fuller for longer,' she says, pointing out that fibre also plays a pivotal role in blood sugar regulation.

The complex structure of wholegrains means the body takes longer to digest them, resulting in slower uptake of sugars from the blood and more stable blood sugar levels. That effect alone can reduce the risk of insulin resistance and type 2 diabetes.

Wholegrains also benefit the gut microbiome. Once undigested fibre reaches the colon, it is fermented by gut bacteria into short-chain fatty acids such as butyrate – a compound shown to improve gut barrier function, reduce inflammation and support healthy immune regulation.

Sadly, wholegrains aren't good for everyone. If you have coeliac disease or gluten intolerance, any grain is off the menu as even small amounts can damage your intestinal lining. And during active flare-ups of Crohn's disease, ulcerative colitis or diverticulitis, high-fibre wholegrains should be avoided as they can worsen symptoms. However, if you have a mild non-coeliac gluten sensitivity, you may be okay to eat a limited wholegrain selection, including quinoa, buckwheat, brown rice and millet.

THE BEST WAY TO GLEAN THE BENEFITS

Different grains contain different types of fibre, and your gut bacteria love variety. So don't just focus on one form, such as wholemeal flour and pasta. That's a good start, but you'll get more benefits if you eat a mix of rye, oats, quinoa, barley and bulgur because each offers unique profiles of prebiotic compounds, minerals and phytonutrients that your gut bacteria will thrive on.

Fortunately, incorporating wholegrains into your diet needn't be complicated. You just need to make a few swaps. Instead of white bread, switch to wholemeal; instead of plain pasta, go for whole-wheat. Oats make an excellent base for breakfast, and cooked brown rice or quinoa can replace white rice at dinner.

And even one portion of wholegrains is enough to see benefits. A 15-year study from Denmark[115] tracked thousands of adults and found that those who consumed the most wholegrains – at least 50g a day – had up to a 34 per cent lower risk of developing type 2 diabetes than those who consumed the least amount of wholegrains. For context, 50g of wholegrains is equivalent to a bowl of porridge or a slice of rye bread – a daily target that's well within reach for most people.

When buying processed foods such as crackers or bread, check the label: ideally the first ingredient should be wholegrain wheat or whole-wheat flour. Where products blend refined grains and wholegrains, a top billing still ensures a good amount of fibre. Oats are typically whole by default, but steel-cut or rolled oats offer more intact fibre than instant varieties.

Sawicki says the greatest health benefits come from consuming around three servings of wholegrains a day. One serving is roughly a slice of bread or a portion of cooked oats, brown pasta or rice. Popcorn, as long as it's not drenched in butter or sugar, also counts as a wholegrain and can be a surprisingly healthy snack – a small bowl provides nearly 3g of fibre. Even swapping your usual mid-afternoon crisps or chocolate for wholegrain crackers and cheese can help.

The idea is to nudge your daily habits in a direction that includes more of the grain, not less. Once you get used to the nutty, fuller flavour of wholegrains, white rice and ultra-soft white bread can seem oddly bland by comparison.

CLEVER WAYS TO BOOST YOUR WHOLEGRAIN INTAKE

★ Mix brown rice with wild rice, quinoa or barley.

★ Make a grain salad base with quinoa, bulgur and farro, and then keep it in the fridge for quick lunches.

★ Mix white and whole-wheat pasta 50:50 until you adjust to the taste.

★ Replace half the white flour in muffins, pancakes or pizza dough with wholemeal flour.

★ Add oat flour (blitz oats in a blender) to banana bread or biscuits for extra nutrition.

★ Toss pearl barley into soups and stews.

★ Switch risotto rice with pearl barley for a creamy risotto or quinoa for 'quinotto'.

★ Use bulgur wheat in place of couscous or make tasty bulgur wheat salads such as tabbouleh.

just one thing

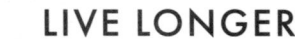

LIVE LONGER

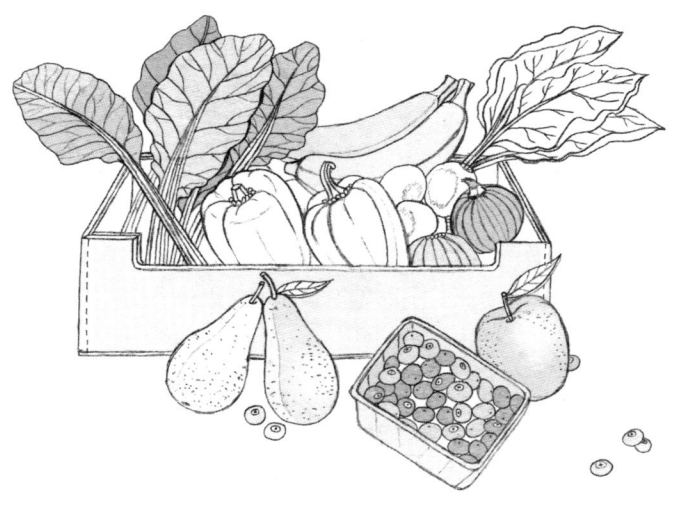

switch sugar
for fruit

How to do it: Swap out sugary snacks and opt for fruit instead.

Why do it? This change can help to lift your mood and boost your memory, may ease cravings to help weight loss, and increase your lifespan.

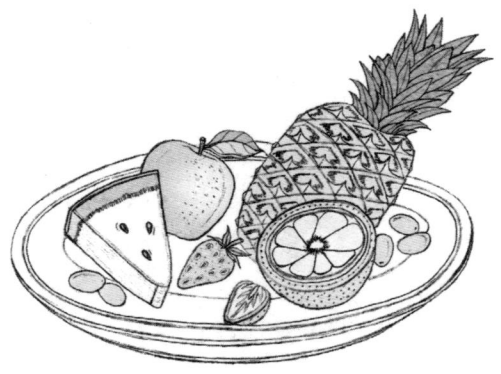

We are a nation of sugar addicts. Sugar is added to so many of the processed foods we eat (yoghurts, cereals, biscuits, bread, baked beans and ketchup) that our brains have become wired to crave the rush of feel-good hormones it provides. As a result, most of us eat more than twice the recommended levels of sugar.

According to the NHS, adults should be eating no more than 30g of 'free sugars' a day. 'Free' means sugars that are easily absorbed by the body, such as the refined sugar you stir into your tea or sprinkle on your strawberries – and which is commonly found in processed foods and drinks. 'Free sugars' also include the naturally occurring sugars found in honey, syrups and fruit juices. Whole fruit doesn't count because the sugars in fruit are naturally contained within the cell walls and the fibre slows absorption to prevent rapid spikes in blood sugar levels. It is surprising how quickly all this sweetness adds up. A glass of apple juice or a shop-bought smoothie can contain nearly 30g of free sugars, which is your full day's allowance. Even savoury processed foods are high in sugar – a jar of ready-made pasta sauce, for instance, can have as much as 7g per portion.

The problem is, our high-sugar diets leave us vulnerable to weight gain, increased risk of type 2 diabetes, heart disease and tooth decay. Eating high levels of sugar can even contribute to inflammation and high blood pressure, as well as affecting our mood and energy levels.

But the studies[116] show that cutting back on sugar – even a little bit – can really be worth it, not only for your teeth and waistline, but in so many other ways. For example, we know that cutting down on free sugars could lift your mood. A 2015 study[117] involving nearly 70,000 women found the lower the levels of added sugars in their diet, the lower their chances of depression. And eating less free sugar could also boost your memory. An Australian study of 4,000 people[118] found that those who drank less than one sugary drink per day had a bigger total brain volume and scored higher on memory tests compared to those who consumed more.

Not only that, but cutting down on sugar, especially sugary drinks, could help you live longer. A huge study[119] looked into the long-term effects of sugary drinks by following nearly 120,000 health professionals in the USA for over 30 years. They found that, the fewer sugary beverages people consumed, the less likely they were to die prematurely from all causes.

TRY WHOLE FRUIT INSTEAD

As anyone who has a sweet tooth knows only too well, the real challenge when you try to stop eating sugary junk food is that you'll sometimes get cravings for something sweet that are hard, if not impossible, to resist. That's where fruit comes in – it tastes sweet, but it is so much better for your health. Switching a sweet snack for a piece of fruit really can help reduce those sugar cravings.

Although fruit does contain sugar in its natural form, that sugar is bound up with fibre, which makes a big difference to how quickly the sugar is absorbed and processed by your body (ideally you should eat the fruit whole, rather than just drink fruit juices, which don't contain as much fibre). Research shows that eating more fibre may even reduce sugary cravings.[120] The other important thing to note is that fruit, particularly the skin, also contains lots of vitamins and flavonoids, which help feed the good bacteria in your gut. For instance, kiwi fruit is a surprisingly good source of vitamin C (90mg per 100g) compared to strawberries (60mg) and even oranges (53mg). Dark fruit such as blueberries, blackberries, cherries, plums and black grapes are rich in health-giving polyphenols.

That 2015 study mentioned earlier (see page 171) found that the women who regularly ate fruit had a lower risk of depression, which suggested a simple swap can deliver a double whammy when it comes to boosting mood. In fact, swapping out your free sugars for some whole fruit comes with a long list of health benefits. As well as improving your microbiome, it may also boost your memory.

Dr Evelyn Medawar from the Max Planck Institute in Germany has been looking at the ways in which swapping sugar for whole fruit can impact our gut microbiome and subsequently our brains: 'Eating a lot of added sugar comes with a lot of implications for the body,' she explains. 'It will cause a spike in glucose which leads to a spike in insulin. And over time, these spikes can lead to insulin resistance, which changes how our body reacts to food, and this can result in more fat being deposited around the body.'

But eating sugar as fruit, she says, is different: 'The fibre in the fruit slows the digestion time and the subsequent metabolic response,' she says. That's why eating a whole apple (skin and all) is better for you than drinking apple juice or an apple-based smoothie. Dr Medawar's research shows one explanation for this is the impact of fibre on our gut microbiome. Her laboratory studies show that eating too much free sugar swells the population of sugar-loving (unhelpful) bacteria in your gut, which then get together to send out difficult-to-resist signals to persuade you to eat more free sugar. 'We found a precise and distinct pathway from the gut acting upon neurons in the brain of the mice in our study, creating a specific preference for sugar,' she says. So those tiny microbes can actually influence the food choices we make.

Conversely, when you eat a piece of fruit, the fibre is very much welcomed by the helpful populations of gut microbes, who use it as fuel for the many important functions they perform on our behalf. Now her studies have shown we can actually dial down cravings for unhealthy foods through eating more fibre. 'It's a very hot topic at the moment!' says Dr Medawar. Her team conducted quite an extensive randomised controlled trial[121] and asked half the volunteers to increase their fibre intake and then measured their food cravings after two weeks. The group which consumed 30g of inulin (which is a prebiotic fibre compound) per day experienced reduced cravings compared to the group eating the placebo powder. 'We measured brain activity to see whether any changes in the reward network were connected to the gut microbiome,' she says, 'and we were very excited to see changes in brain activity levels after just two weeks.'

Her top tip is to reduce consumption of high-sugar foods in your diet. And her second piece of advice is to replace your sweet treats with high-fibre whole fruit. So, when you are hit by a sugary craving, why not try snacking on fruit instead?

THE NUTRITIONAL POWER OF FRUIT

★ **Apple** (skin on) 4.4g fibre plus vitamin C, potassium and polyphenols

★ **Banana** 3g fibre plus potassium, magnesium and vitamins B6 and C

★ **Blueberries** (150g) 4g fibre plus antioxidants and vitamins C and K

★ **Grapes** (10) 0.6g fibre plus resveratrol and vitamins C and K

★ **Mixed berries** (frozen 150g serving) 6g fibre plus vitamin C, antioxidants, folate and manganese

★ **Orange** 3g fibre plus vitamin C, folate, thiamine and potassium

★ **Peach** 1g fibre plus niacin, potassium and vitamins C and A

★ **Pear** (skin on) 6g fibre plus vitamin C, potassium and antioxidants

★ **Raspberries** (150g) 8g fibre plus vitamin C, manganese and antioxidants

★ **Strawberries** (150g) 3g fibre plus vitamin C, folate and antioxidants

just one thing

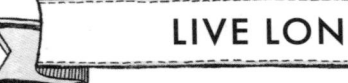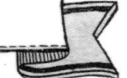

LIVE LONGER

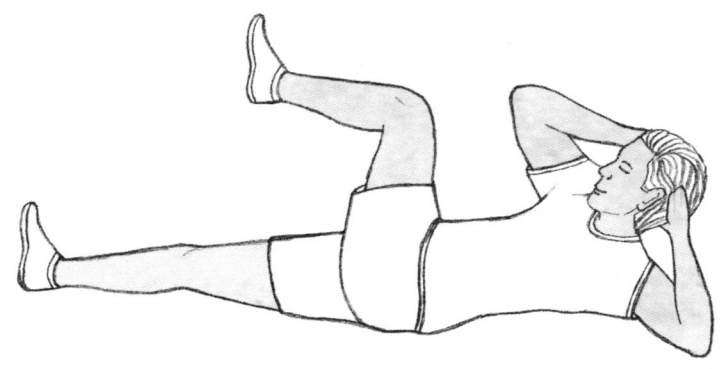

hit the HIIT

How to do it: Aim to do two HIIT (high-intensity interval training) workouts a week.

Why do it? HIIT increases cardiovascular fitness, may boost memory and cognitive performance, and could even extend your lifespan.

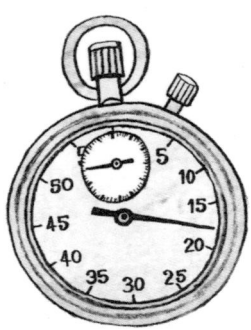

If you're not a fan of exercise, you may be encouraged to hear that sometimes, less really can be more. We know exercise is good for us, but many people struggle to find the time to fit enough in, let alone meet the official recommendations for 150 minutes of moderate activity per week. So it's great to know that there's one form of activity, called HIIT or high-intensity interval training, which can not only burn more calories in a considerably shorter time, but can also build your muscles and boost your brain power.

HIIT is a training technique that involves short bursts of intense exercise – whether you're walking, running, swimming or cycling – followed by brief recovery periods. The idea is, you work flat out for 30–60 seconds, pause to catch your breath, then push hard again for 30–60 seconds, repeating the pattern multiple times.

And studies increasingly show that a HIIT workout that's done and dusted in less than 15 minutes could be as effective as spending much *much* longer doing traditional exercise.

Professor Martin Gibala is professor of kinesiology at McMaster University in Ontario, Canada, and the author of many fascinating experiments comparing HIIT and conventional exercise. He is very impressed by the way HIIT improves cardiovascular fitness. 'Your heart becomes a better, stronger pump,' he says. 'Your stroke volume goes up too – that's the amount of blood that is ejected with each beat of your heart. We also see improvements in insulin sensitivity and markers of blood sugar control after various types of high-intensity interval training.' All these markers are consistent with a reduced risk of dying from all causes – particularly the common killers of cardiovascular disease and type 2 diabetes.

CHANGES IN CELLS

One small study Professor Gibala conducted back in 2006[122] compared two weeks of sprint interval training with more traditional, moderate-intensity continuous training. For the study, the HIIT group was asked to do six 30-second all-out sprints with a few minutes of recovery between each. Their total training per session was about 25 minutes. The other group spent two hours on continuous moderate exercise at each session.

Professor Gibala and his team then measured the activity of mitochondria (organelles that are the power units in our cells) in muscle. Mitochondria tend to become less effective as we age. The higher your mitochondrial content the better, as this is associated typically with improvements in your blood sugar control. Any form of exercise has been shown to be effective at helping to remove old mitochondria and stimulating the growth of new ones, but Professor Gibala's study shows that HIIT is particularly effective at doing this.

In another study,[123] volunteers were asked to do a HIIT protocol that involved cycling at maximum intensity for four lots of four minutes. They did this three times a week. After three months, the participants had not only improved muscle mass and strength, but they had increased their mitochondrial activity by up to 70 per cent.

In their 2006 study, Professor Gibala and his team found very similar improvements in muscle responses between the two groups. Both groups saw an increase in markers for mitochondrial capacity despite the fact that the sprint group was only giving about 20 per cent of the total exercise and time commitment.

He is convinced it is the intensity that is key – you are better able to give maximum effort when you know that's only required for a few seconds. He likens the effect to pushing the accelerator on a car. 'Traditional moderate-intensity exercise is a bit like pushing halfway down on the accelerator. This causes your fuel levels to slowly drop. But high-intensity exercise is more like stomping on the pedal. It will cause the fuel gauge to drop very quickly.' This brief but extreme impact on the body triggers a process of cellular remodelling which is most definitely a good thing. This is what enhances our physiological capacity.

Not only does HIIT give better results at the cellular level than other forms of exercise, but it may also be better for your brain. Research has shown it can boost memory and cognitive performance in both young and older adults more than moderate exercise can. That's because, when we exercise at a higher intensity, our muscles produce lots of lactate as fuel for our cells. Lactate travels to the brain, where it boosts the production of a chemical called brain-derived neurotrophic factor (BDNF). This is a hormone that stimulates the production of new brain cells and helps protect existing brain cells.

Not only that, but HIIT could also help you live longer than other forms of exercise. A Norwegian study[124] randomised 1,500 adults to either doing HIIT or moderate exercise, and they were asked to stick to this protocol for five years. It turned out that HIIT had the biggest impact on both quality of life and fitness. It also led to the biggest reductions in death from all causes.

HOW TO HIIT

Whether it's HIIT or anything else, do check with your doctor if you're starting a new exercise regime or if you have previous injuries. Professor Gibala suggests taking it gently at first: 'If you're just starting, just aim to get out of your comfort zone so your heart rate is a little higher, or you're maybe a little more out of breath,' he says.

There are many different kinds of HIIT protocols, and the principles can be applied to anything you're doing, whether that's walking, jogging, cycling, swimming or even dancing. To make it HIIT, you just have to work hard for 10–60 seconds, then rest for 10–60 seconds and repeat the cycle a few times. You can introduce intervals of more vigorous intensity into almost any form of exercise. For instance, there's evidence[125] to show that in many people just brisk walking, particularly if it's uphill, is enough to achieve benefits. Stair-climbing can be fantastic. Even if your only physical activity is walking around the block at night, as simple as it sounds, just try picking up the pace between a few lamp posts, and then back off to your normal pace for a few – injecting a few bursts of speed.

'HIIT incorporates a broad range of exercise intensities,' says Professor Gibala, 'and the degree of intensity is a very personal choice. Most people can perform vigorous exercise in a safe manner – the key is making the intensity vigorous for you.' He says it is a big misperception that for HIIT to be effective you need to go all out: 'Aim to work at a challenging pace, but you don't need to go all-out as hard as you can go during these efforts.'

'High intensity means vigorous effort as opposed to moderate or light effort,' he says, 'so devise your own 10-point scale where one is completely sedentary or lying on the couch, and 10 is sprinting from extreme danger or running as hard as you can to save your child from an oncoming car. For the sort of vigorous exercise you need to be thinking about for HIIT, aim for about seven or eight on your 10-point scale.'

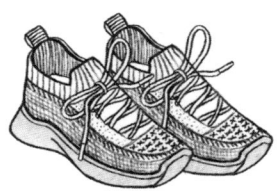

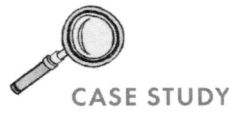

CASE STUDY

Suzanne, an NHS worker from Northern Ireland

'I work full-time as the team leader for a group of 12 nurses, and with a husband and two children of primary-school age, my exercise time is limited! I try to get out on a 20-minute walk every day at lunchtime, but sometimes I have to miss my walk if I'm snowed under with other commitments.

'I've been trying to infuse HIIT protocols on my normal walk, picking up the pace every three minutes. It's actually easier to just walk a bit faster and I like to think I'm getting a much better workout in a shorter amount of time. After my walk, I have noticed that I'm in a better mood. I've enjoyed feeling energised and motivated to get on with the rest of my day. I've also tried running on the spot for five one-minute intervals. That's quite hard if I'm honest and it did feel as if I'd completed a full workout class even though it was only 15 minutes.

'On the days I do HIIT, I've noticed that I slept better that night. I'm more energised, and I feel positive to be doing something good for my health.'

BEGINNER-FRIENDLY HIIT PROTOCOL

This 10-minute circuit is a great HIIT taster for someone who isn't used to exercising. It involves five rounds of brisk walking followed by slow walking (recovery).

1. **WARM UP** your muscles and circulation by marching on the spot or walking slowly around a room for 2–3 minutes, rolling your shoulders and swinging your arms.
2. **SET A TIMER** and walk briskly for 20 seconds, swinging your arms.
3. **RETURN** to a slow walk for 70 seconds to recover your breath.
4. **REPEAT** five times.
5. **YOU CAN GRADUALLY BUILD** your endurance by extending the brisk walk to 30, then 40, seconds and ultimately one minute, reducing the duration of the slower recovery walk.
6. **AS YOU GET FITTER**, you can increase the challenge by walking uphill (or putting a treadmill on an incline) and by pushing yourself progressively harder during the intense intervals.

Not only does HIIT give better results at the cellular level than other forms of exercise, but it may also be better for your brain. Research has shown it can boost memory and cognitive performance more than moderate exercise can.

just
one
thing

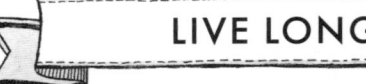

LIVE LONGER

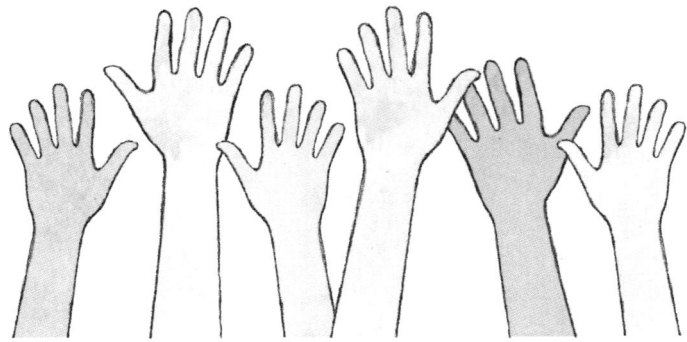

try volunteering

How to do it: Sign yourself up for volunteering once a month.

Why do it? It may boost mood, reduce stress, lower cholesterol, reduce chronic inflammation and slow the ageing process.

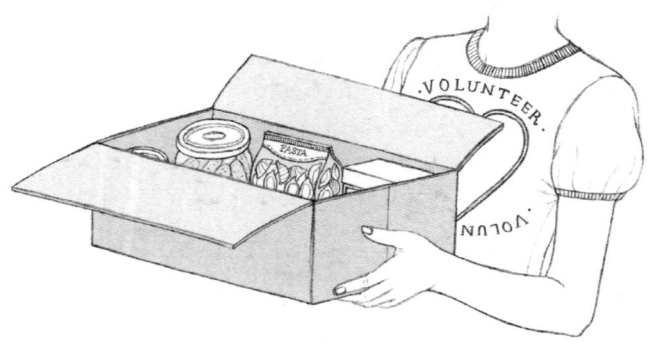

Volunteering isn't just good for the community – it's good for you, too. Studies show it has benefits for both mental and physical health. Whether you're offering time, skills or simply a listening ear, the process of giving back creates a sense of purpose and connection, but it may also be good for your heart in a completely literal sense by lowering cholesterol and reducing chronic inflammation (a body-wide immune response, often initially triggered by infection, injury or irritation, but persisting for months or years).

The science really does back this up. For example, one study[126] involving more than 7,000 older Americans found that those who volunteered spent 38 per cent fewer nights in hospital. A follow-up study in 2020[127] found that volunteering for as little as two hours a week was linked to a lower risk of an early death and an improved sense of wellbeing, compared to people who don't regularly volunteer.

One way that volunteering may help extend healthy life is by lowering blood pressure. In an American study,[128] researchers followed older adults for four years, none of whom had high blood pressure to begin with. Those who volunteered for about four hours a week were 40 per cent less likely to have high blood pressure at the end of the study. So do people who volunteer tend to be healthier and more health conscious anyway? Or does volunteering have a direct effect on our health, perhaps by reducing stress?

MIND–BODY CONNECTION

Dr Edith Chen from Northwestern University, in the USA, has investigated the ways in which helping others can lower chronic inflammation and strengthen the health of our hearts. She and her team tested the hypothesis that volunteering is beneficial for people's physical health by recruiting high-school students[129] and randomly assigning half of them to weekly volunteering (helping out at an after-school club for younger children) for one semester, while the other half continued with their usual habits. The team studied the participants' physical health, measuring obesity, cholesterol and inflammation, both before and after the volunteering programme was completed. They found that the students in the volunteering group had lower levels of obesity and on all other counts compared to the students who weren't allocated to the volunteering project.

Dr Chen says: 'We believe the psychosocial benefits of volunteering translate into physiological and physical health effects through a sort of mind–body relationship – proving that our mental state can impact our physical health.'

In her study, the volunteering group showed the biggest decreases in negative mood and also in inflammation. 'This suggests that volunteering helps to put people in a better mood and this links to lower levels of inflammation,' she says. The volunteering group also showed greater increases in empathy (developing a greater concern for and understanding of other people's feelings), and interestingly, she says, 'The participants with the greatest increase in empathy during the intervention period also showed the greatest decreases in inflammation.'

The team saw this by measuring the inflammation markers interleukin-6 and C-reactive protein. Studies have shown that people with higher levels of these biomarkers are at greater risk for a variety of diseases like heart disease, stroke and diabetes later in life.

Dr Chen believes any type of volunteering elicits health benefits but speculates that the effects might be larger if your volunteering has a sociable aspect to it, because that way you also get to enjoy positive interaction with other people and you get to experience feedback. There are observational studies that suggest giving your time has a greater health impact than merely making a money donation, she adds.

Some research suggests that your motive matters. To be truly effective, your volunteering should be generous and heartfelt. In the study where researchers asked older people to record their motives for volunteering, they found that those who volunteered tended to live longer. But the twist was, this was only true if the volunteers genuinely *wanted* to help others, rather than just doing it to make themselves feel better. This suggests altruism may be an important factor in how volunteering benefits our health.

And it's never too late to start. In fact, one 2025 study[130] found that regular volunteering helps to slow the ageing process, reducing your risk of chronic health conditions, particularly once you hit retirement.

Although the participants in Dr Chen's studies were encouraged to volunteer once a week, she says there's no optimal commitment – the most important factor is that volunteering becomes a regular habit. 'Everyone has busy lives, and it's not always feasible to volunteer once a week but doing it every other week, or even once a month, is still good,' she says. 'It's the regular, consistent volunteering as opposed to a one-time action that has the potential to benefit your health and wellbeing most.'

HOW TO START VOLUNTEERING

1. START WITH YOUR INTERESTS. Think about what you're passionate about or where you'd like to make a difference, whether it's supporting people with mental health challenges, helping animals, working in a charity shop, tackling food poverty or conserving the environment. Once you've considered what you personally enjoy doing, look for organisations that do that work and check out their websites for volunteer opportunities.

2. BE REALISTIC ABOUT YOUR TIME. You don't need to commit hours every week. Many organisations offer flexible, one-off or remote opportunities. If your schedule is tight, consider micro-volunteering: short, often online tasks that still make a difference, such as proofreading or mentoring.

3. LOOK LOCAL. Check with your local volunteer centre or council-run community network or volunteer services. Libraries, hospitals, food banks and sports clubs often rely on volunteers and welcome new offers of help.

4. TRY A NATIONAL DATABASE. Websites like Doit Life (www.doit.life/volunteer; the UK's national volunteering database), Reach Volunteering (https://reachvolunteering.org.uk; a UK charity that provides volunteering opportunities in community organisations such as food banks, schools, refugee support and mental health projects) or Volunteering Matters (https://volunteeringmatters.org.uk; a UK-wide charity that creates structured volunteering programmes) allow you to search opportunities by location, cause and skill level. National bodies such as the Royal Voluntary Service, British Red Cross, National Trust, Wildlife Trusts, NSPCC, Girlguiding and Scouts also rely heavily on volunteers and have flexible roles suitable for beginners.

5. ASK YOUR EMPLOYER. Many companies support volunteering through paid volunteer days or partnerships with charities, so it's worth checking what's available through your workplace.

6. DON'T BE AFRAID TO TRY SOMETHING NEW. Volunteering can be a great way to gain skills and meet new people. If your first experience doesn't feel like a good fit, try another. The right role will feel rewarding, not overwhelming.

just one thing

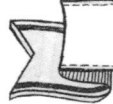 LIVE LONGER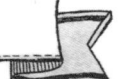

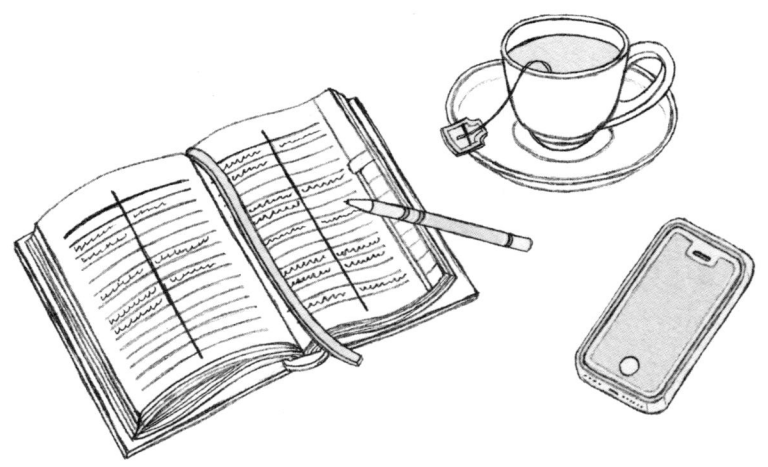

reach out

How to do it: Say hello to a stranger, chat with a neighbour or send a random 'Hello, how are you?' text.

Why do it? This can extend life expectancy by encouraging better sleep and heart health, protecting your brain from ageing, reducing dementia risk and strengthening immunity.

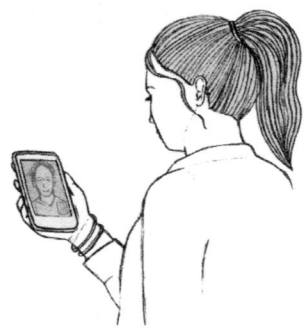

Human connection is good for your heart and your sleep, and it can even influence how well you recover from illness. In fact, there's plenty of research to show that cultivating strong social ties really can have a big impact on your health, and there are lots of very good reasons to aim to be a little more sociable – even if you do it in a small way.

For example, one of the longest human studies ever carried out began in the 1930s when researchers recruited more than 700 men from Harvard and the surrounding area.[131,132] They were then followed for decades. Some, like the future US President John F Kennedy, became rich and famous, but others led less illustrious lives. The researchers consistently found it wasn't fame, money, social class or IQ that kept people happy and healthy throughout their lives, it was having satisfying relationships.

Good friendships are so important, they might even protect your brain from the ravages of age. When scientists investigated super-agers – people in their 80s who had the memory skills of people several decades younger – they found they had more positive social relationships in their lives than others who were not fortunate enough to live so long.[133]

And a Swedish study[134] which followed 1,200 older people discovered that those living alone or without close social ties were at greater risk of developing dementia. But reassuringly even occasional visits with friends kept the risk down.

It's not just about having a select few close relationships. It seems you'll benefit most if you have a wide range of social contacts. This means not just friends and family, but also neighbours, work colleagues and others in the wider community. In one rather macabre study,[135] scientists took nearly 300 healthy volunteers and deliberately infected them with a common cold virus. They found the volunteers with a rich diversity of social ties were four times less likely to develop a cold than those who were less outgoing. And if they did get a cold, they didn't suffer from annoying symptoms quite as much.

A LONG AND SOCIABLE LIFE

Social connections may even help you live longer, too. When scientists analysed results of nearly 150 different studies, which included over 300,000 people,[136] they found those with the strongest social relationships had the greatest life expectancy.

Professor Pamela Qualter from the University of Manchester is an expert on the importance of social relationships. She says: 'We now know that social relationships really matter, and we've shown again and again that loneliness has an impact on health, on sleep, and longer term it has an impact on cardiovascular health, too.'

Her studies show that casual relationships also count: 'The seemingly superficial relationships you might have with someone who always gets on the same train as you, or the barista who makes your coffee each morning, actually matter quite a lot,' she adds. 'It's all about feeling connected.'

Professor Qualter studied the specific impact of interacting with neighbours.[137] She asked half the participants to do a kind act for someone else each week for four weeks and the other half to go about their normal social interactions. The results showed that actively taking part in this kind challenge saw loneliness levels reduce over time. 'Making connections definitely seems to release endorphins,' explains Professor Qualter, 'it helps you feel better about yourself, and about the community in which you live.' Her findings corroborate other research that shows that volunteering (see page 183) makes people feel a lot better in themselves, increases life satisfaction and increases mental wellbeing.

She believes a text or email also has benefits in terms of social connection: 'I think we all realised during the pandemic that social media plays an important role in enabling us to connect. And I think during very stressful times, it's really important to send out text messages and take every opportunity to show others that you're thinking about them.'

However, it is clear from the science that physical touch remains very important. 'Studies show touch releases certain brain hormones that make us feel good,' Professor Qualter says. 'Being close to people we care about can stimulate the release of the hormone oxytocin.' Ensuring we get enough physical connection in our everyday lives will release all-important feel-good oxytocin.

HOW TO REACH OUT

Professor Qualter is keen to encourage us all to boost our social connections if we can. 'Start with something simple like a nod of the head, a smile, or saying "hello" to someone you pass in the street or at the bus stop,' she says. 'Just think about different ways you can engage with other people.'

Then, she suggests, aim to build that bond by offering support to a neighbour – perhaps offer to put their bins out. 'You just need to engage in a way that makes you feel you're part of a community. But the best route is to simply start talking to people, start getting out and engaging with others. And if you can't get out of the house and do that, do it on social media.'

So why don't you try reaching out a bit more? Ring that friend you haven't seen for ages, organise a video call with someone who's moved abroad or even just go and knock on your neighbour's door. You may find that other people are just as pleased to connect with you as you are with them. And there are lots of health benefits to be gained for you and for them.

WAYS TO BOOST YOUR SOCIAL LIFE

1. LEVERAGE EXISTING INTERESTS AND HOBBIES. Look for clubs or groups centred around your hobbies, sports or other interests. In these groups, you are more likely to meet like-minded individuals.

2. SIGN UP FOR A CLASS. Whether it's cooking, dancing, learning a new language or some kind of activity, classes provide structured opportunities to interact with others.

3. VOLUNTEER. Find organisations or causes you care about and volunteer your time. This is a rewarding way to meet people who share your values.

4. ATTEND COMMUNITY EVENTS. Local festivals, farmers' markets, workshops and other community gatherings offer casual settings to meet new people.

5. BE OPEN TO NEW CONNECTIONS. Practise initiating conversations and making introductions, and don't be afraid to strike up conversations with strangers.

6. JOIN ONLINE GROUPS. If you aren't very mobile, join online forums or groups related to your hobbies and participate in discussions.

just one thing

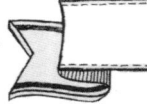 LIVE LONGER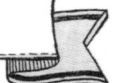

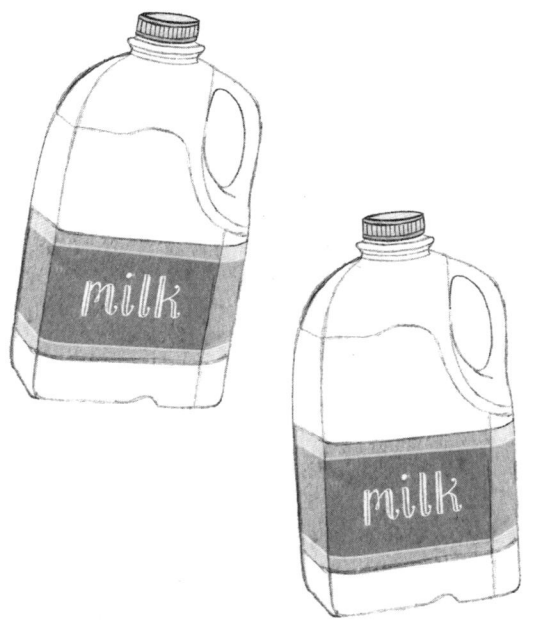

lift weights

How to do it: Incorporate some weightlifting into your exercise regime twice a week.

Why do it? Weightlifting can improve mood and immunity; benefit heart, brain and bone health; and slow the pace of ageing.

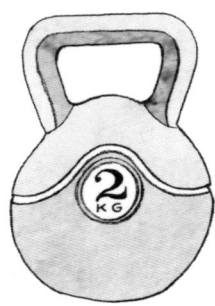

You might think that weightlifting will give you bulging biceps or muscly thighs, but adding a bit of weightlifting or resistance training into your regular exercise regime could have an impact on your health that's more far-reaching than merely sculpting a gym-honed silhouette.

Increasingly, research is showing that challenging and strengthening your muscles by working against the resistance of weights, bodyweight (press-ups, for example), resistance bands or machines for just a few minutes twice a week can confer some remarkable health benefits.

In recent years, we have become really focused on weight and body fat, and the link between obesity and disease, but an American study[138] found good muscle mass to be one of the strongest predictors of longevity, even more than weight or body mass index (BMI, a measure of your weight in relation to your height). Researchers followed 3,600 men and women over the age of 50 for a decade, and found that those who had more muscle mass were at a lower risk of death from all natural causes.

Specialists in exercise physiology know that regular weightlifting can boost your metabolism because muscle burns more calories at rest than fat, so the more muscle you have, the greater your calorie burn. That, in turn, can help you manage your weight. Also, because active muscles draw glucose out of the blood, weight training can help to balance blood sugar levels. This can help protect you against type 2 diabetes.

BODY BENEFITS

Studies have even shown that strength training can enhance your immunity. One study[139] looked at cells called neutrophils, which form part of the immune system's first line of defence. When your body is trying to fight a virus or infection, these cells are deployed to surround and engulf pathogens. When the researchers compared women who were mostly sedentary with those who regularly did resistance training, they found the strong women had far more active neutrophils, indicating that their immune system was more robust.

Strength training will build bone health and help protect against conditions such as osteoporosis, but it may help to reverse ageing at a cellular level, too. In one small but fascinating study,[140] scientists asked a group of older men to undertake two sessions of resistance training twice a week, and then compared them to a group of younger men before and after a six-month period. After just six months they found that resistance training influenced gene expression – which means it changes which genes are turned on or off – to help improve health, muscle function and metabolism, which would normally decline with age. It can essentially 'reprogramme' gene activity to a more youthful state.

MEMORY BOOST

And finally, strength training can do very good things for your brain power. It might seem counterintuitive to think that building brawn can also build your brain and protect your white matter, but it's true! Dr Teresa Liu-Ambrose is professor of physical therapy at the University of British Columbia in Canada. She is a keen exponent of strength training to help maintain muscle strength and bone health as we get older, and is confident that maintaining muscle mass helps you reduce your risk of chronic conditions such as type 2 diabetes and heart disease. But her novel research shows that strength training can also directly impact both your brain function and brain structure to improve your memory, as well as more complex cognitive abilities such as decision-making.

She and her team compared the brain-boosting benefits of strength training in two groups of over-65s – one group who were in good health and one group with cognitive impairment.[141] 'In both groups, we found that strength training had benefits for cognitive function,' she says. Her studies showed that, with strength training, people were better able to remember things and specifically saw improvements in 'associative memory' – the ability to remember someone's face and name some time after first meeting them. 'We also found that, with strength training, people had better executive functions, meaning that they were able to make the appropriate decision based on the circumstance presented to them,' she adds.

Dr Liu-Ambrose believes there are multiple pathways by which exercise brings benefits for cognitive and brain health. One is the way exercise stimulates release of brain chemicals, such as brain-derived neurotrophic factor (BDNF) and insulin growth factor (IGF), which ensure the survival of neurons and, crucially, promote the growth of new neurons. But one more recent discovery is the role of specialised hormones called 'myokines'. She explains that these hormones are produced in the muscles and released when muscles contract. 'Current evidence suggests once you release these hormones they travel throughout the body and go to different organs and tissues, where they jump-start a variety of chemical processes,' she says. 'When you engage in exercise, these hormones cross the blood–brain barrier and arrive in the brain, where they enhance other chemicals, such as BDNF, which is like a kind of fertiliser for the brain, helping to preserve brain cells.'

Her research marks a real shift in how we think about the ways in which exercise impacts the brain: 'Traditionally, we've been very focused on what's released in the brain and not on peripheral mechanisms,' she says, 'but the knowledge about this muscle–brain crosstalk really enriches our understanding of the role that muscles play in bringing about benefits when we exercise.'

STARTING ON WEIGHTLIFTING

There's no doubt it is definitely worth adding a bit of weightlifting to your exercise regime. The NHS recommends that all adults (whatever your age) engage in muscle-strengthening activities on at least two days per week, in addition to 150 minutes of aerobic activity. But do check with your doctor first if you're starting a new exercise regime or you have any previous injuries.

Complete beginners can start with simple bodyweight exercises such as squats, lunges or wall presses, or with light resistance work using free weights, weight machines or resistance bands. You'll find explanations of key movements at www.nhs.uk (type 'strength exercises' into the search bar) or take a look at 'Three key strength-building exercises' on pages 200–1.

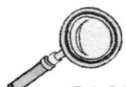

CASE STUDY
Jenny from Manchester
'The only exercise I routinely do is housework, but I was happy to try a bit of weightlifting, especially as I don't need special equipment. I did bicep curls using a bottle of milk as a weight, calf raises (holding on to a countertop and lifting myself up on to tiptoes) and weighted squats with a rucksack full of books on my back. I ran through the exercises (three sets of 10) every day for 15 minutes while watching TV. I found it easier to fit into my busy schedule than I expected. I particularly liked the fact that I didn't have to get changed or get to a gym.

'To be honest, I never imagined myself lifting weights, but I have definitely noticed improvements. I feel physically and mentally stronger and my posture has improved.'

THREE KEY STRENGTH-BUILDING EXERCISES

1. BICEP CURLS

Using a bottle of milk as a weight (a 2-litre bottle weighs about 2kg when full, so start with the bottle half-empty), stand or sit and grasp the bottle with one hand, with your palm facing forwards (underhand grip). Keeping your elbow close to your side, slowly bend your arm to bring the bottle up towards your shoulder, squeezing your bicep as you lift. Hold for one second at the top, then slowly lower to the start position. Aim for 10 repetitions then switch arms. Repeat three times for each arm.

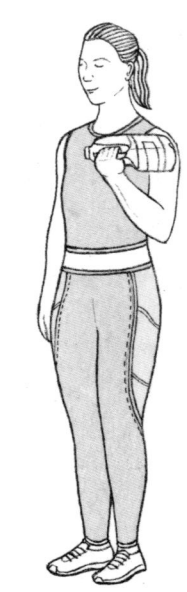

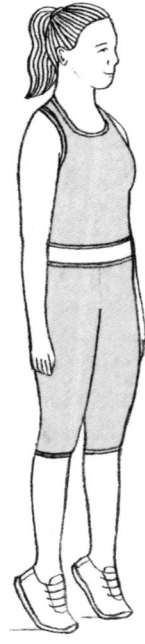

2. CALF RAISES

Stand facing a countertop with your feet hip-width apart and toes pointing straight ahead. Slowly raise your heels off the ground so you're standing on the balls of your feet, hold at the top for one second, squeezing your calf muscles, then slowly lower. Aim for three sets of 10 repetitions.

3. WEIGHTED SQUATS

Fill a backpack with books or cans and wear it high on your back (start with light weights and increase the weight as you get stronger). Stand with your feet shoulder-width apart, your toes pointing slightly outwards. Keeping your chest up and your shoulders back, push your hips back as if sitting in a chair, bending your knees until your thighs are parallel to the floor. Keep your weight in your heels and your knees tracking over your toes. Push through your heels to stand back up, squeezing your buttock muscles at the top. Repeat three sets of 10 repetitions with a short break in between each set.

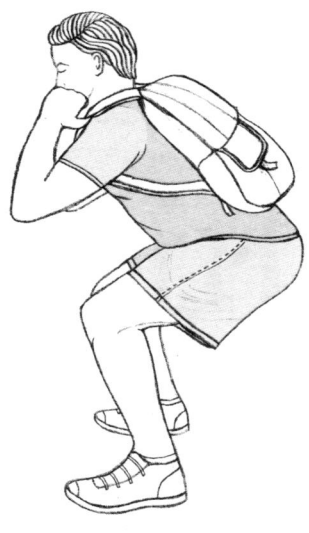

just one thing

KEEP YOUR HEART HEALTHY

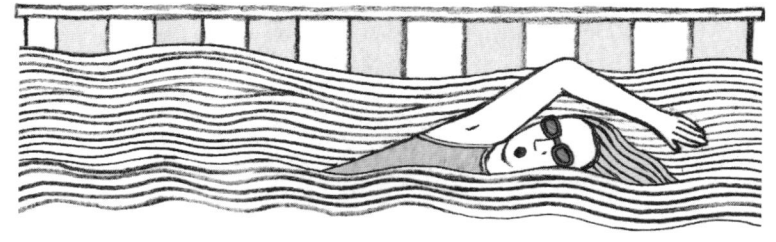

go swimming

How to do it: Swim for 20–30 minutes three times a week.

Why do it? Regular swimming may protect against heart disease and help boost brain function.

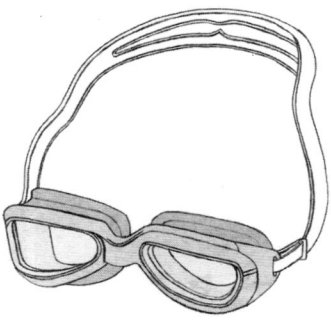

Swimming has unique benefits over other forms of exercise. Not only is it gentle on the joints and accessible to all ages, but it also provides a powerful workout for both body and brain. Whether you're doing steady laps or simply marching up and down in the shallow end, being in water means you will be engaging many of your major muscle groups and gaining surprising cardiovascular and cognitive benefits.

While any form of exercise is better than none, swimming appears to have unique properties that go beyond what you might gain from walking, running or cycling on dry land. It's not just about the resistance of the water, or the cooling effects that allow you to train for longer. Swimming enhances vascular health in ways other activities don't, potentially helping to stave off heart disease and cognitive decline.

Let's begin with longevity. In a landmark study[142] conducted by researchers at the University of South Carolina, more than 40,000 men aged 20–90 were tracked over 13 years. The results were striking: swimmers had a significantly lower death rate than those who didn't exercise at all – and even compared with runners and walkers, swimmers were 50 per cent less likely to die from all natural causes.

Swimming also appears to offer neurological benefits. In one animal study, just seven days of swim training was enough to improve memory in rats. And while rodent studies can't be taken as definitive evidence for humans, similar effects are beginning to emerge in human trials. A small New Zealand study,[143] for example, found that just 20 minutes of swimming enhanced brain function and even led to slightly faster reaction times.

EXPANDING BLOOD VESSELS

But what makes swimming so uniquely beneficial? Professor Hirofumi Tanaka, an exercise physiologist at the University of Texas at Austin, believes the answer lies in the way water-based activities interact with our cardiovascular system.

'Heart disease is not really a disease of the heart,' he explains. 'It is a disease of the blood vessels and arteries. A blockage in an artery can cause a heart attack; a blockage in the brain can cause a stroke.' He continues: 'Most people think arteries are just pipes that carry blood, but they also have another function – to cushion and buffer the pulsations of the heart. When arteries become stiff with age, those pressure waves travel straight to the brain or other organs, where they can cause damage.'

That's where swimming comes in. Research led by Tanaka has found that three months of regular swimming can significantly reduce arterial stiffness – more so than walking, running or cycling. The mechanism is not fully understood, but it appears that exercising in water causes a beneficial shift in blood flow and pressure, making arteries more elastic and better able to absorb the heart's pulsations. To test this theory further, Tanaka compared the effects of cycling on land and cycling underwater. Remarkably, those who pedalled in a submerged environment saw greater reductions in vascular stiffness and bigger improvements in cardiovascular markers.

There is also growing evidence that exercising in water boosts blood flow to the brain. One of Tanaka's studies looked at Nordic walking (see page 215) – a full-body workout involving ski-like poles – and compared its effects on land and in water. Because the technique utilises muscles in the arms and torso as well as the legs, it activates large areas of the brain and scans show regular Nordic walking can enhance cognitive function. But when participants performed the same arm-swinging, big-stride movements underwater, results were even more pronounced. After three months, those who regularly tried Nordic walking in water not only saw improvements in vascular health but also measurable gains in brain performance.

Part of the beneficial effect of swimming may be mechanical. Unlike upright exercises such as jogging or cycling, swimming takes place in a horizontal position, which may make it easier for blood to reach the brain. In addition, the hydrostatic pressure of water naturally encourages blood flow towards the core, enhancing circulation to vital organs including the brain.

TIME TO GET WET

Swimming is also low impact, making it ideal for those with arthritis, joint pain or limited mobility. 'Because swimming is a non-weight-bearing activity, it's excellent for older adults,' Tanaka says. His research has shown that swimming regularly can reduce joint pain, improve functional ability and lower risk factors for vascular disease.

As little as 20–30 minutes of swimming, three times a week, is enough to see real changes, Tanaka says. And you don't have to be doing a slick front crawl or energetic butterfly action to benefit. Even walking vigorously up and down the shallow end will provide resistance and pressure that can improve circulation and challenge your muscles.

'The important thing is to keep moving in the water,' Tanaka adds. 'You will be working against the resistance of the water and therefore using more muscle groups than you would on land and stimulating blood flow in a way that seems to benefit both body and brain.'

With the UK boasting a strong network of local authority pools, swimming is one of the more affordable and accessible ways to get active. Whether you're a lapsed swimmer or a complete beginner, it might be time to take the plunge.

GETTING INTO THE SWIM

If it's been a while since you last swam – or if you're entirely new to it – the key is to begin gently and build up gradually. Most local authority pools offer adult-only sessions, some of which are designated for beginners or slower swimmers. Ask about confidence classes or refresher lessons, which can help ease you back into the water with guidance on technique and breathing.

Start by setting modest goals: 15–20 minutes of continuous movement in the water is enough to begin with. You don't have to swim laps. Water walking, slow breaststroke or even moving your arms and legs while holding on to the pool's edge all count. Over time, aim to build up to 30 minutes, two to three times a week.

TIPS FOR SWIMMERS

1. DON'T WORRY ABOUT SPEED OR DISTANCE. Focus on good form and consistency.

2. USE EQUIPMENT. Floats, kickboards and pool noodles can help build strength and improve technique.

3. TRY A CLASS. Water aerobics or aqua-fit sessions offer structure, motivation and low-impact cardiovascular benefits.

4. TAKE REST BREAKS. Swim a length, then pause for 30 seconds before continuing.

5. DRINK PLENTY OF WATER. You still sweat in the pool, even if you don't notice it.

just
one
thing

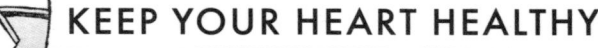

KEEP YOUR HEART HEALTHY

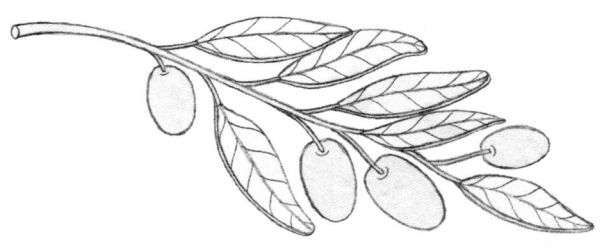

drizzle olive oil

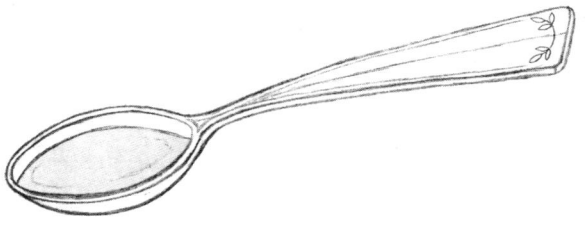

How to do it: Consume 2 tablespoons (around 30ml) of olive oil a day.

Why do it? It may lower blood pressure, help protect the heart, reduce inflammation and preserve brain function.

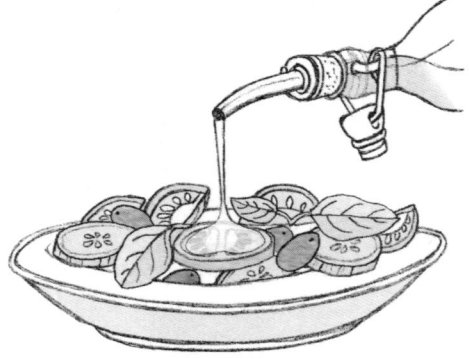

The Mediterranean diet has long been hailed as a gold standard for healthy living, with research consistently linking it to a lower risk of heart disease, stroke and cognitive decline. At the very heart of this diet is olive oil. It's not just a culinary staple but a nutritional powerhouse, particularly in its extra virgin form.

While both regular and extra virgin olive oil are high in heart-healthy monounsaturated fats, it's the extra virgin variety that has been attracting serious scientific attention. Cold-pressed and minimally processed, extra virgin olive oil (EVOO) retains more of the beneficial compounds found in olives – especially polyphenols. These plant-derived antioxidants are thought to play a key role in olive oil's health-promoting effects, from lowering chronic inflammation to improving the function of blood vessels – two key processes in the development of heart disease.

A recent Spanish study[144] involving more than 12,000 people found that those who consumed around one and a half tablespoons of extra virgin olive oil a day were nearly 50 per cent less likely to die from cardiovascular disease than those who used refined or ordinary olive oil. This association did not hold for non-virgin oils, suggesting the polyphenols in EVOO may provide the extra protection. However, a 2022 meta-analysis[145] found that olive oil in any form was effective at reducing blood pressure, although EVOO had the edge thanks to its higher antioxidant load.

However, polyphenols don't tell the full story. Olive oil is also a rich source of oleic acid, a monounsaturated omega-9 fatty acid that appears to have significant anti-inflammatory properties. Dr Bill Mullen, a nutrition researcher at the University of Glasgow, has been studying the effects of olive oil on heart health. 'Oleic acid is certainly known for having anti-inflammatory effects, and we're pretty sure a lot of chronic diseases start with inflammation,' he says. 'If it does have that effect, it probably helps protect the arterial walls by preventing plaque build-up.'

Dr Mullen's research goes beyond traditional measures such as blood cholesterol or blood pressure. He and his team have pioneered an approach that looks for protein biomarkers in urine that reflect an individual's risk of coronary artery disease. 'Cholesterol isn't always a reliable predictor,' he explains. 'Someone with high cholesterol can have good heart health, while another with low cholesterol can still suffer a heart attack.'

In one study,[146] Mullen and colleagues gave two groups of healthy volunteers 20ml (just under two tablespoons) of olive oil each day – one group received extra virgin, the other refined. Urine samples were collected at three and six weeks to look for changes in disease markers. Surprisingly, both groups showed a statistically significant reduction in heart disease risk, despite participants already being healthy at baseline.

'EVOO might have additional polyphenols that confer other benefits, but when we look purely at coronary artery disease biomarkers, the type of olive oil didn't seem to matter,' Mullen says. That's encouraging news for those put off by the higher cost of extra virgin varieties – any olive oil appears to be better than none.

Cooking with olive oil is also safe, despite persistent myths to the contrary. While it's true that oil heated beyond its smoke point can degrade and produce harmful compounds, olive oil's smoke point is higher than often assumed – around 190–220°C, depending on the type. For most home-cooking, including roasting, sautéing and light frying, olive oil is perfectly suitable. 'It's a very stable fat,' says Mullen. 'As long as you're not reusing the oil repeatedly at very high temperatures, it's actually quite safe – and the health benefits outweigh any minor risks from cooking.'

BRAIN TONIC

Beyond the heart, olive oil could also be a powerful brain tonic, too. A small but intriguing study[147] looked at 25 older adults with mild cognitive impairment – a condition often seen as a precursor to dementia. Participants were randomly assigned to consume either regular or extra virgin olive oil daily (30ml, or roughly two tablespoons) for six months. Both groups experienced improvements in memory tests, but those consuming EVOO also showed better brain connectivity on MRI scans and improved integrity of the blood–brain barrier – a crucial defence against harmful substances.

'This suggests that compounds in extra virgin olive oil may help preserve brain function as we age,' says Mullen. 'And if oleic acid is good for the arteries in your heart, it stands to reason it's also good for arteries in the brain.'

Olive oil's anti-inflammatory powers are also drawing attention from researchers interested in cancer, autoimmune conditions and metabolic disorders. Chronic inflammation (a persistent, long-term immune system response) is now understood to be a driver not just of heart disease and Alzheimer's but of a wide range of conditions from type 2 diabetes to bowel cancer. A recent review of 30 clinical studies[148] found that daily consumption reduced levels of two key inflammation markers – interleukin-6 and C-reactive protein. 'The evidence is stacking up,' says Mullen. 'There's really no downside to using olive oil liberally – whether that's drizzled over salad, stirred into soup or used as your go-to cooking fat.'

Even the flavour has its perks. EVOO has a distinctive peppery taste – a sign of its rich polyphenol content – that enhances dishes without the need for added salt or processed dressings. So, how much should you aim to consume? Most studies suggest that around one to two tablespoons a day offers a meaningful health boost. Use olive oil, ideally EVOO if you can afford it, in place of your other oils. Look for 'cold-pressed' and 'unfiltered' on labels for the highest polyphenol content. Store away from heat and light to preserve freshness.

WAYS TO GET YOUR DAILY OLIVE OIL FIX

1. DRIZZLE OVER ROASTED VEGETABLES. Once your vegetables are cooked, add a tablespoon of EVOO before serving. Heating during cooking can degrade some of the beneficial compounds, so post-roast drizzling retains more polyphenols.

2. SWAP FOR BUTTER IN MASH AND BAKING. Olive oil gives mashed potatoes a creamy texture and subtle flavour – just use around two-thirds of the amount of butter you'd typically add. Olive oil can also replace butter in many cake and muffin recipes.

3. MAKE YOUR OWN DRESSING. Combine EVOO with lemon juice, Dijon mustard, garlic and herbs for a zingy, heart-healthy salad dressing that's free from additives.

4. ADD TO SOUPS AND STEWS. A swirl of oil just before serving enhances flavour and brings extra anti-inflammatory power.

5. DIP AND ENJOY. Use good-quality olive oil as a dip for crusty wholemeal bread, with a dash of balsamic vinegar or sprinkle of za'atar.

just
one
thing

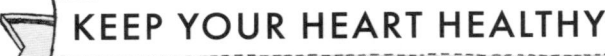

KEEP YOUR HEART HEALTHY

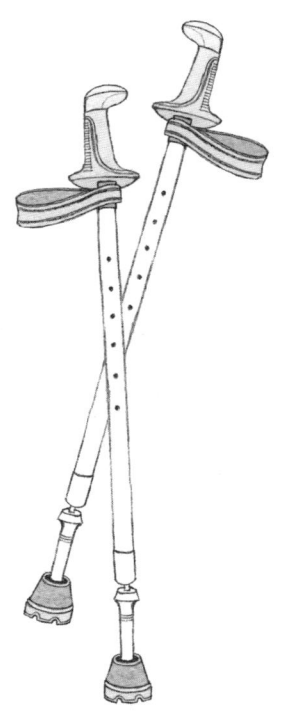

go Nordic
walking

How to do it: Invest in a pair of poles and make every walk a Nordic walk.

Why do it? It may reduce the risk of cardiovascular disease and can improve fitness, fat loss, flexibility and strength, while helping to preserve brain power and slow cognitive decline.

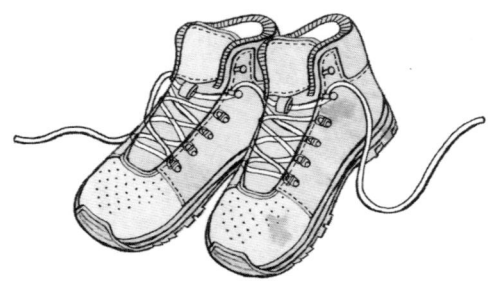

Nordic walking, a rhythmic form of exercise where you walk with specially designed poles to engage the arms and upper body, is fast gaining popularity as an effective way to improve both physical and mental health. Originating in Finland in the 1930s, Nordic walking was first developed as a sport by cross-country skiers to help them stay fit in the off-season. Today, it's catching on everywhere from suburban pavements to city parks and coastal promenades.

Unlike ordinary walking, which works the muscles in the lower body, Nordic walking engages the whole body. A regular stroll might use around 40 per cent of your muscles, but Nordic walking puts demands on up to 90 per cent of muscles, including those in your arms, shoulders, chest, back and abdomen, as well as your legs.

The technique is relatively simple: you walk briskly, using poles to push off the ground with each step, propelling yourself forwards while maintaining an upright and open posture.

Crucially, this added muscle engagement doesn't just make you feel more energised – it actually leads to meaningful changes in your body. In one 12-week study of older women with osteoporosis,[149] participants who practised Nordic walking three times a week experienced significant improvement in knee strength and functional performance. Their balance, walking speed and confidence all improved too, with researchers crediting the full-body engagement of the activity for their gains.

Another key benefit is calorie burn. Nordic walking has been shown to burn 20–40 per cent more calories than regular walking, even when speed and distance are kept the same. That's because the body is working harder overall, with more muscles involved in every stride. For those who want to boost their cardiovascular fitness or lose weight without putting extra strain on their joints, it's an appealing alternative to jogging or high-impact workouts.

In a six-month Italian study,[150] 38 middle-aged adults were randomly assigned to walk briskly three times a week, one group with poles and the other without. While both groups saw improvements in fitness, only the Nordic walkers experienced a significant reduction in body fat. The researchers attributed this to the greater muscle involvement and higher energy expenditure required when using poles.

Nordic walking also appears to offer therapeutic benefits. A trial involving 80 people with chronic lower-back pain[151] showed that those who took up Nordic walking for an hour, two to three times a week for just four weeks, experienced a marked reduction in pain. Compared with a control group who continued their usual routines, the Nordic walkers also showed improvements in flexibility, strength, cardiovascular fitness and – perhaps most strikingly – a 23 per cent improvement in self-reported mental wellbeing.

It's not just in studies linked with back pain that the mental health effects are being noticed. Many practitioners of Nordic walking report a positive mood boost simply from getting outside and walking with purpose, rhythm and good posture. There's also emerging evidence that Nordic walking may offer neurological benefits, particularly for older adults. Engaging the upper and lower body together, in a rhythmical and coordinated way, appears to stimulate the brain in a manner that some neuroscientists now describe as 'neuroprotective'. Activities that require coordinated movement, attention and balance may help to preserve executive function and delay cognitive decline, and Nordic walking ticks all of these boxes.

BENEFITS FOR CARDIOVASCULAR DISEASE

Perhaps the most compelling research to date comes from a recent trial led by Dr Jennifer Reed, a cardiologist and researcher at the University of Ottawa Heart Institute. She and her colleagues wanted to test whether Nordic walking could benefit people with established cardiovascular disease – people for whom every gain in fitness counts. Patients were randomly assigned to one of three types of exercise[152] over 12 weeks: Nordic walking, moderate to vigorous continuous training (such as using an elliptical trainer or jogging) or high-intensity interval training (HIIT). All three groups saw improvements in heart health, but the Nordic walkers saw the biggest gains in what's known as functional capacity, which was measured by how far they could walk in six minutes. An improvement of 54m is considered to be clinically meaningful. The traditional cardio group improved by 48m, and the HIIT group by 51m, but the Nordic walking group improved by an impressive 77m.

Dr Reed believes that the success of Nordic walking lies in its comprehensive impact on the body. 'It strengthens the upper and lower body, improves posture and confidence, and increases walking speed,' she explains. 'You're also improving your aerobic fitness, your strength and your endurance simultaneously.'

Other studies support this view. There is evidence that Nordic walking improves blood pressure, cholesterol and glucose levels, as well as aiding weight management. It offers a way to increase oxygen uptake and metabolic rate without increasing mechanical stress on the joints, making it an excellent option for those with arthritis, obesity or mobility limitations.

For those who are sceptical about picking up poles, Dr Reed says the results speak for themselves. 'Nordic walking is a great form of physical activity, and any physical activity is important for managing and preventing chronic disease,' she says. 'We all have the ability to modify 80 per cent of our risk for cardiovascular disease. Nordic walking is one tool that's especially accessible and effective. Anyone who can walk can benefit. That's because the poles both support you and propel you.'

Nordic walking is scalable, social and suitable for people of almost any age or fitness level. It tones muscle, strengthens the heart, improves mood and posture, and even burns more calories than jogging, all without requiring you to move any faster or further than an ordinary walk.

HOW TO WALK WITH POLES

Nordic walking is not difficult and you can learn the technique from an instructor or from videos online. You can borrow poles or buy your own online. Dr Reed recommends starting slowly, aiming for just a few minutes at a time until the movement becomes natural. 'Once you're comfortable, you can build up to 10 minutes, then 30, and eventually aim for 150 minutes a week,' she says – the level of physical activity recommended for overall cardiovascular health. Try these tips:

★ Start with big strides, letting the poles drag along the ground beside you. When you start to engage the poles, your arms should swing forwards and back in opposition to your legs, as in normal walking.

★ Hold the poles loosely with the glove-like strap around your wrist and keep them pointing diagonally backwards as you walk. Place the poles on the ground in turn on either side of your feet as you walk.

★ As you place each pole on the ground, grip it tightly and push down to propel yourself forwards. After pushing yourself forwards, let go of the handle by opening your hand.

★ Take big 'heel then toe' strides, squeezing your buttock muscles. Allow your upper body to rotate as you swing your arms, walking in a fluid motion. Maintain an upright posture with your shoulders relaxed.

★ You can 'double pole' (using both poles together) to get up or down steep sections.

just one thing

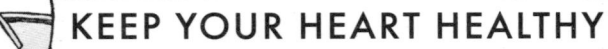

KEEP YOUR HEART HEALTHY

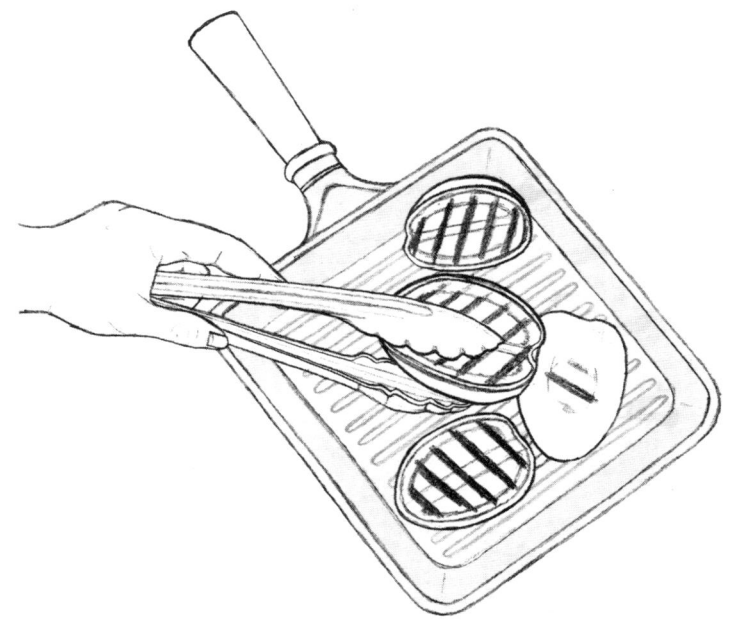

cook tomatoes

How to do it: Add a portion of tomatoes (preferably cooked) to your diet five times a week.

Why do it? This could improve cholesterol levels and reduce inflammation as well as the risk of prostate cancer.

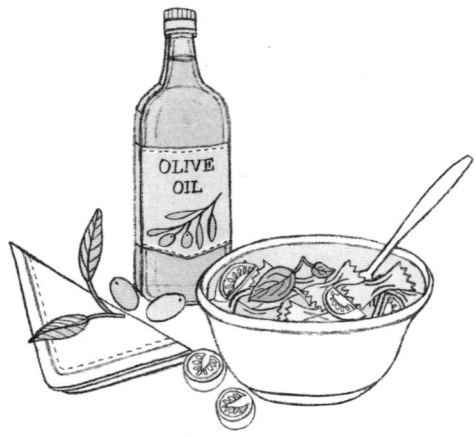

There is much to admire about the tomato: its bright acidity, juicy flesh and refreshing flavour make it a staple of summer salads and Mediterranean diets. But although raw tomatoes are rich in vitamin C, potassium and folate, when cooked their full health potential is truly unlocked.

At the heart of the tomato's nutritional power is lycopene, a vivid red pigment which acts as a potent antioxidant that can help to neutralise harmful free radicals in the body. These are the unstable molecules that can damage cells and contribute to ageing and disease. Although you get a hit of lycopene when you eat raw tomatoes, the compound becomes significantly more bio-available when tomatoes are cooked. That's because heat breaks down the fruit's thick cell walls, releasing the lycopene and making it easier for the body to absorb.

Tomatoes are technically fruit because they contain seeds and develop from the ovary of a flower. Yet they have long been treated as a vegetable in culinary circles. When tomatoes first arrived in

Europe from the Americas in the 16th century, they were viewed with suspicion. Their vibrant red colour was seen as alluring but potentially toxic. Centuries on, they are one of the most consumed fruits in the world. They are linked with a range of health benefits, from improved cholesterol profiles to better skin health. Evidence suggests that they may even lower the risk of certain cancers.

Modern research suggests that the humble tomato can do much to support cardiovascular health. In a review of six studies,[153] researchers found that consuming a large glass of tomato juice daily over six weeks was linked with an improvement in blood fat (lipid) profiles. Participants showed reductions in LDL (low-density lipoprotein, aka 'bad') cholesterol and increases in HDL (high-density lipoprotein, aka 'good') cholesterol.

The benefits of tomato juice may go beyond the heart. In a small Greek study,[154] athletes who drank tomato juice instead of energy drinks during periods of strenuous exercise experienced quicker muscle recovery and showed reduced markers of inflammation in their blood. Lycopene, once again, appears to be a key factor.

CANCER PROTECTION

There is growing interest in the role of cooked tomatoes in reducing the risk of prostate cancer. Several observational studies[155] have found that men who regularly consume tomato products such as sauces and pastes have a lower incidence of prostate cancer. Prostate-specific antigen (PSA) levels, a key marker of prostate health, also appear to benefit.

So how exactly does this one antioxidant confer such a wide range of benefits? According to Professor Richard van Breemen of Oregon State University, lycopene appears to help reduce oxidative stress, which is a type of cellular damage that plays a role in ageing and many chronic diseases. His research shows that certain organs, such as the prostate, may be more vulnerable to this kind of stress.

Over the last 20 years, there has been quite a bit of research into lycopene's anti-cancer properties, and van Breemen has focused much of his interest on the potential protective benefits of lycopene on prostate cancer, which is the second major cause of death among men in the Western world. He began his clinical work with tomato sauce. 'At first, we wanted to see if a realistic dietary amount of lycopene could reach the blood and the prostate,' he says, 'so we recruited a group of men who were at risk for prostate cancer. We prepared meals, mainly pasta dishes, with tomato sauce which could deliver around 30 milligrams of lycopene per day.' His studies showed that the lycopene was getting through to the right place – levels doubled in the blood and the prostate. 'We also observed a measurable reduction in oxidative stress,' he adds.

This matters because, as van Breemen explains, 'Many organs in the body have an extremely efficient way to check the DNA in the nucleus of the cells and repair it, but the prostate is less able to repair DNA damage, and this damage can accumulate over time. Lycopene can help prevent that initial DNA damage, reducing the load that the body has to bear and the extent of the repairs that have to be made,' he says.

COOKING IS KEY

For those seeking to make the most of the benefits of tomatoes, cooking is key. Whether you sauté tomatoes for a pasta sauce, roast them for a rich soup or blend them into juice, it is the heat which breaks down the fruit's structure and makes lycopene more accessible.

What's more, pairing cooked tomatoes with a source of fat, such as olive oil, further boosts absorption. 'Lycopene is what we call an oil-soluble vitamin,' says van Breemen, 'so to help extract it from the plant as we eat it, a little bit of oil like olive oil goes a long way.'

Eating a tomato salad might give you 5 or 10mg of lycopene, but cooking and blending your tomatoes yields much more: 100g of tomato sauce will deliver roughly 50mg of lycopene.

For both women and men, studies show skin health may also benefit from eating a diet rich in cooked tomatoes. One small trial[156] gave participants 40g of tomato purée with olive oil to eat every day for 10 weeks and found their skin resilience improved – the incidence of sunburn dropped by 40 per cent. Another small study[157] found 40g of tomato purée with olive oil helped to protect the skin against DNA damage and increased levels of pro-collagen, which helps to keep skin firm and youthful looking.

Despite its potent activity, lycopene is safe. 'You cannot overdo it,' van Breemen says. It's a bonus that tomatoes are so versatile and affordable that it's not hard to add more into your diet. Not everyone enjoys the acidity of raw tomatoes, but the mellow sweetness that develops with cooking can be more palatable. For those looking to boost their lycopene intake without radically altering their diet, small adjustments can make a significant difference.

A bowl of tomato soup, a spoonful of tomato purée stirred into a stew or even a glass of low-sodium tomato juice, can all contribute to your lycopene levels. Add tomato purée to casseroles, blend it into smoothies or spread it over wholegrain toast as a base for other toppings. And yes, even pizza has its place, provided it's topped with a rich tomato base and enjoyed in moderation.

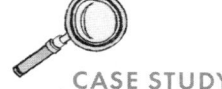

CASE STUDY

Chris, a recently retired IT manager from Nottinghamshire
'I wouldn't say I'm the biggest tomato eater in the world. Tomatoes do slip into my diet, but they are not something I focus on eating. But I battle with high cholesterol and recently I've had a raised PSA level (which could indicate prostate problems). Fortunately, in my case, everything was clear and there was nothing to worry about. But it's given me a heightened awareness.

'So I was happy to stock up on tomatoes: fresh, tinned, passata, a ready-made soup and some posh tomato ketchup. I always thought the healthiest way of eating a tomato was in a salad but tipping tinned tomatoes into a bolognaise sauce is much more appetising. We ended up making pasta bakes, soups, a vegetable risotto and even a tomato and prawn curry – and actually found it quite easy to add five portions of cooked tomatoes over the week.

'I'll still get my cholesterol and PSA measured every year. And hopefully, increasing my tomato intake will have a positive impact.'

just one
thing

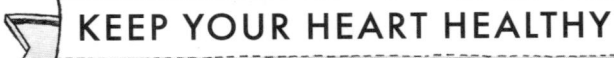

KEEP YOUR HEART HEALTHY

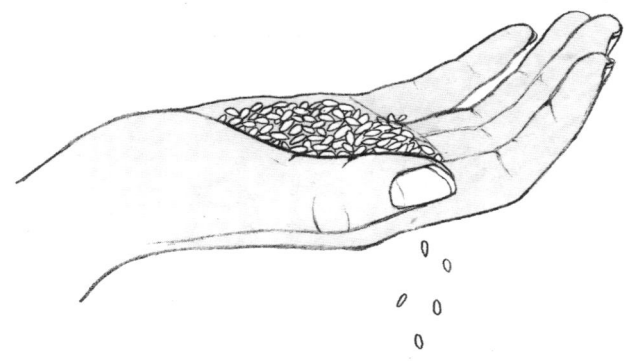

sprinkle flaxseeds

How to do it: Add 2 tablespoons of ground flaxseeds to your diet each day.

Why do it? It may smooth skin, lower blood pressure and inflammation, and improve cholesterol profiles, thereby reducing the risk of strokes and heart attacks.

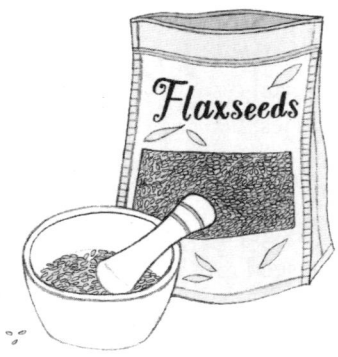

Flaxseeds, also known as linseeds, may be small, but their nutritional profile is mighty. These glossy brown or golden seeds have been eaten for centuries, but in recent years, scientists have begun to uncover just how good they are for our health. From lowering blood pressure to smoothing your skin, flaxseeds are emerging as a simple – and evidence-backed – addition you can make to your daily routine.

The seeds are rich in fibre, plant protein, lignans and alpha-linolenic acid (ALA), an omega-3 fatty acid that offers a powerful mix of health benefits that target many of the most common chronic conditions, from high blood pressure to type 2 diabetes.

Much of the early evidence for flaxseeds has been focused on heart health. One of the leading researchers in this area is Dr Grant Pierce from the University of Manitoba in Canada, who has spent decades investigating the cardiovascular effects of flaxseeds. 'Flax is unique,' says Dr Pierce. 'It contains three beneficial compounds: ALA, which is anti-inflammatory; fibre, which helps reduce cholesterol; and lignans, which are powerful antioxidants.'

Taken together, he says, these components act on multiple systems in the body – reducing oxidative stress, improving cholesterol profiles and lowering inflammation, all of which are risk factors for heart disease. 'Very few foods contain all three of these compounds, and certainly not in the quantities found in flaxseeds.'

One of the most compelling studies led by Dr Pierce[158] was a year-long, double-blind (where neither the participants nor the researchers know who is receiving the active treatment and who is receiving a placebo), randomised controlled trial involving patients with peripheral arterial disease – a condition that causes blockages in the arteries, leading to leg pain, high blood pressure and increased cardiovascular risk. Half the participants were randomly assigned to consume 30g of ground flaxseeds daily, disguised in muffins, bagels, pasta and snack bars. After 12 months, those in the flaxseed group experienced an average 15mmHg drop in systolic blood pressure – a change that, in public health terms, could translate to a 50 per cent reduction in strokes and heart attacks.

'The blood pressure changes were dramatic,' says Dr Pierce. 'In fact, they were among the largest seen in any dietary intervention, including the Mediterranean diet or salt reduction.' The flaxseed group also saw cholesterol levels fall by around 10 to 15 per cent – enough to cut cardiovascular risk by a further 20 per cent.

The underlying mechanism, according to Dr Pierce, involves the ALA in flaxseed blocking an enzyme known as soluble epoxide hydrolase (SEH). This, in turn, leads to a rise in molecules that not only reduce inflammation but also dilate blood vessels – creating a dual-action effect that appears to lower blood pressure and protect against vascular damage.

It's not just heart health that benefits. Flaxseeds have also shown promise in improving blood sugar regulation. In a small study published in 2020,[159] participants who consumed 30g of ground flaxseeds per day had lower blood glucose levels across the day compared to those who didn't eat flaxseeds. This effect is likely to be due to the high fibre content, which slows the absorption of sugar into the bloodstream. Their rich fibre content also helps keep bowel movements regular and may relieve constipation.

Flaxseeds are also very good for your skin. In a small German study,[160] women with sensitive skin who consumed flaxseed oil daily for 12 weeks reported reduced skin irritation and improved hydration and smoothness. Researchers suspect the fatty acid content, particularly ALA, plays a role in strengthening the skin barrier and reducing inflammation.

Although most of the research has focused on cardiovascular and metabolic health, scientists are beginning to explore flaxseeds' potential role in preventing cancer, particularly hormone-sensitive types such as breast and prostate cancer. Lignans, which are present in particularly high amounts in flax, have weak oestrogenic properties which means they may modulate hormone metabolism in ways that reduce risk. While evidence is still emerging, it adds to the growing picture of flaxseed as a valuable addition to the modern diet.

HOW TO TAKE YOUR FLAXSEEDS

For best results, flaxseeds should be ground before eating. Whole flaxseeds can pass through the digestive tract undigested, meaning you miss out on many of their beneficial nutrients. A coffee grinder works well for blitzing the seeds fresh, and once ground, they can be stored in the fridge for several weeks. 'You'll know if they've oxidised,' says Dr Pierce. 'They'll start to smell fishy.'

Importantly, flaxseed appears to be safe for most people and doesn't seem to lower blood pressure excessively in those with normal readings. In Dr Pierce's studies, even participants with healthy blood pressure didn't see any adverse effects – only those with high readings benefited from a significant drop. 'It seems to work like an adaptogen,' he says. 'If you need the help, it gives it. If you don't, there's no harm.'

The recommended daily dose is 1–2 tablespoons of ground flaxseeds, but research suggests even lower amounts may still provide measurable benefits. Having said that, it's wise to start on very small amounts if you have digestive sensitivities as too much fibre can cause bloating, gas or diarrhoea in some people. The omega-3 content also has mild blood-thinning properties, so large amounts may interact with anticoagulants, and the phytoestrogens might make them unsuitable if you have hormone-sensitive breast cancer.

MEET YOUR FLAXSEED TARGETS

1. SPRINKLE ON FOOD. One of the easiest ways to include flaxseeds in your diet is to grind them and sprinkle them over your food. Their mild, nutty flavour makes them a natural addition to porridge, cereal, yoghurt, smoothies or even savoury dishes such as soups and salads.

2. SUPER-CHARGE YOUR BAKING. Simply add 1–2 tablespoons of ground flaxseeds to baked goods like banana bread, muffins or granola bars. It blends in well and adds a subtle texture and nutritional boost. If you're adding a lot (more than 2–3 tablespoons), you may need to slightly increase the liquid in your recipe to maintain a soft texture. Used whole or ground, flaxseeds hold up well to baking temperatures and retain most of their benefits.

3. SUBSTITUTE PART OF THE FLOUR. If a baking recipe calls for 200g of flour, you can replace up to 50g with ground flaxseeds. This adds fibre, healthy fats and a mild nutty flavour without drastically changing the texture.

4. USE AS AN EGG REPLACEMENT. Mix 1 tablespoon of ground flaxseeds with 3 tablespoons of water, stir well, and leave to sit for 5–10 minutes until it forms a gel. This 'flax egg' works well in cookies, muffins, pancakes and brownies.

WILL A FLAXSEED CAPSULE WORK JUST AS WELL?

You can buy flaxseed capsules which contain flaxseed oil extracted from the seeds. The capsules are a concentrated source of omega-3 fatty acids, which may be useful for heart health and reducing inflammation. However, you won't be getting the benefit of the fibre, the lignans (plant phytoestrogens with antioxidant effects) or protein.

just one thing

KEEP YOUR HEART HEALTHY

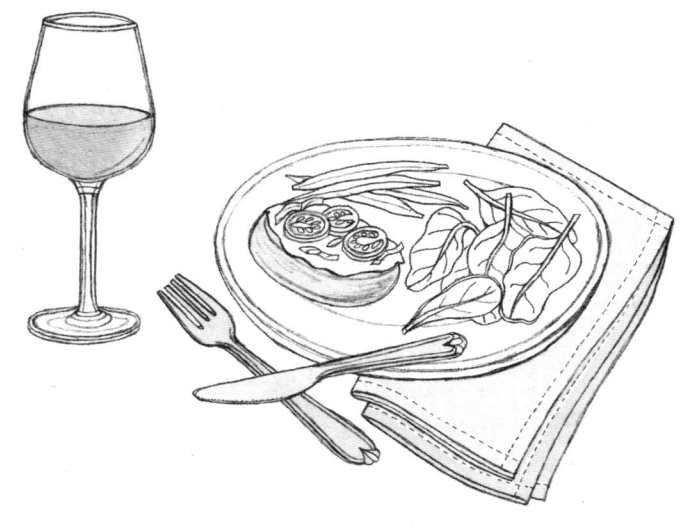

switch to red wine

How to do it: Swap your usual tipple to red wine (in moderation).

Why do it? Switching to red wine may protect the heart, help to regulate blood sugar and boost the diversity of gut bacteria.

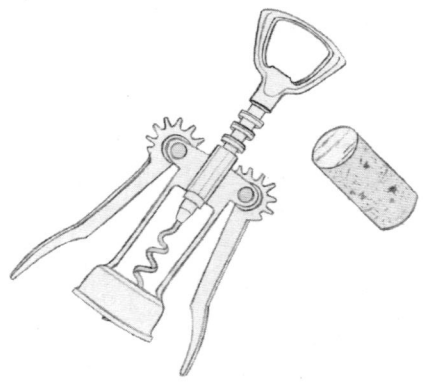

There's no escaping the truth: alcohol, in general, is not good for us. It's linked to everything from liver disease and cancer to poor sleep. If you don't drink, there's no compelling reason to start. But for those who do enjoy the occasional tipple, there may be a case – albeit a modest one – for reaching for a glass of red wine.

Not only does red wine taste delicious, but it may also offer some intriguing health benefits. Mounting research suggests that, in small quantities and consumed with food, red wine could help protect your heart, regulate blood sugar and even boost the diversity of your gut bacteria. The root of red wine's potential health halo lies in its high concentration of polyphenols: beneficial plant compounds found in the skins and seeds of red and black grapes. These polyphenols are known for their antioxidant and anti-inflammatory properties, and they may also support the health of our arteries and microbiome.

THE FRENCH PARADOX

The idea that red wine might be good for us was first floated in the 1980s, when researchers noticed something curious: despite eating a diet relatively high in saturated fat, the French population had surprisingly low rates of coronary heart disease compared to Americans. This observation became known as the 'French paradox' and launched a wave of speculation that regular wine consumption – particularly red – might be the secret.

At the time, it was an appealing narrative: the notion that a pleasurable indulgence could double as a health tonic. But as scientific understanding deepened, the idea began to look less robust. It now seems likely that the French advantage has more to do with their overall diet – rich in vegetables, legumes, fruit and oily fish – and smaller portion sizes, than with wine.

Still, red wine hasn't entirely lost its scientific sheen. In 2015, a group of Israeli researchers conducted a rigorous trial involving 224 people with type 2 diabetes.[161] Participants were randomly assigned to drink a medium glass of red wine, white wine or mineral water with dinner every evening for two years. The wine and water were supplied free of charge, and empty bottles were collected to track adherence.

The results were striking: those who drank red wine experienced modest but measurable improvements in cholesterol levels and blood sugar control. They also reported better sleep quality than the white wine or water groups. Crucially, no significant adverse effects were reported.

A Spanish study[162] went further, showing that red wine consumption may improve insulin sensitivity – meaning the body clears sugar from the blood more efficiently. Timing, too, matters. A recent longitudinal analysis of over 300,000 people[163] found that wine consumed *with* a meal was linked to a 14 per cent lower risk of developing type 2 diabetes. The benefit was lost, however, when the wine was drunk outside mealtimes.

GUT INSTINCTS

One of the more exciting areas of red wine research is its impact on the gut microbiome – the community of trillions of bacteria that reside in our digestive system and are now understood to play a role in everything from immune function to mood.

Professor Tim Spector, an epidemiologist at King's College London and one of the UK's leading experts on gut health, has spent years analysing microbiome data from thousands of people. His findings show that those who drink red wine in moderation tend to have a more diverse microbiome, which is a marker of good health. 'A diverse microbiome is like a thriving rainforest,' he explains. 'It means you've got more species in your gut capable of producing beneficial chemicals to support immunity, metabolism and digestion.'

Interestingly, drinkers of other types of alcohol – beer, spirits, even white wine – do not show the same microbiome benefits. 'Generally, alcohol is detrimental to gut health,' says Professor Spector. 'But red wine appears to be an exception, most likely due to the high levels of polyphenols derived from the grape skins.'

These polyphenols, he says, seem to act as fuel for beneficial gut microbes. While alcohol typically suppresses microbial diversity, red wine appears to foster it – provided consumption is moderate. 'We were able to show that, once you reach three glasses of red wine per day, you start to lose any benefit,' he warns.

For a time, the health appeal of red wine was pinned on a single compound: resveratrol, a polyphenol found in grape skins and touted for its anti-ageing potential. But the latest research suggests that resveratrol is just one player in a much larger orchestra.

'In a single glass of red wine, there could be thousands of different polyphenols and related compounds,' says Professor Spector. 'The beneficial effects are likely to come not from one "magic" molecule, but from the complex interactions between many.' In other words, you can't simply bottle red wine's health potential into a pill.

A DRINK FOR EVERYONE?

So, should we all be drinking red wine for our health? Not necessarily.

If you drink alcohol, do so in moderation and within NHS guidelines. The UK's chief medical officers advise that adults drink no more than 14 units of alcohol per week: roughly equivalent to nine small (125ml) glasses of wine (or four large 250ml glasses). Drinking should also be spread out over several days, with alcohol-free days in between.

Professor Spector agrees that any benefit from red wine comes with caveats. 'The most favourable picture emerges when red wine is consumed in small amounts, with food, and as part of a balanced, Mediterranean-style diet,' he says. 'We're talking about traditional wine glasses – six to a bottle – not the enormous goblets many of us use at home.'

For those who are pregnant, have a history of addiction or liver problems, or are taking certain medications, alcohol of any kind is inadvisable. And those already teetotal should not view red wine as a health supplement in disguise.

But if you already enjoy the occasional glass, there's no need to feel guilty – particularly if you choose red wine, drink it with food and keep it in moderation. You might even be doing your heart, blood sugar and gut a small favour.

HOW TO PICK A POLYPHENOL-RICH WINE

If you're drinking red wine for the potential health benefits, not all bottles are created equal. Polyphenol content can vary dramatically depending on the grape variety, climate and how the wine was made.

Wines made from thicker-skinned grapes – like Cabernet Sauvignon, Syrah (Shiraz), Malbec and Tannat – tend to be richest in polyphenols, especially a sub-group called flavonoids. Wines that are deeply coloured, tannic and full-bodied usually indicate higher levels of these beneficial compounds. Look for traditional, dry reds with minimal sugar, and avoid heavily processed or mass-produced wines, which often contain fewer natural polyphenols.

just
one
thing

BE STRONGER AND FITTER

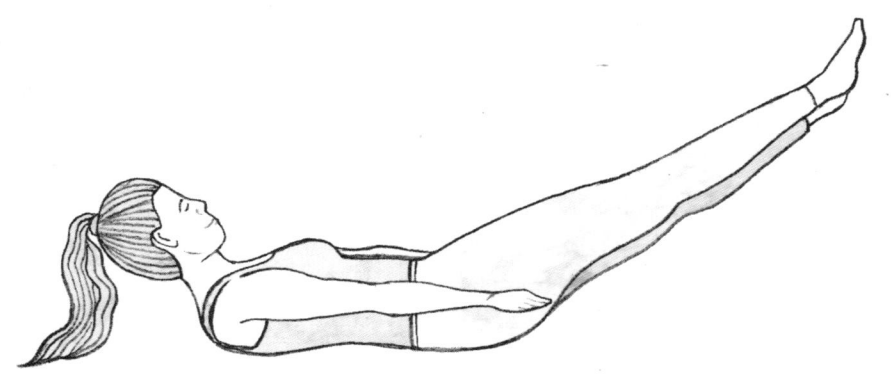

practise Pilates

How to do it: Practise Pilates for 30 minutes, three times a week.

Why do it? Practising Pilates can elevate mood and improve core strength, posture and balance.

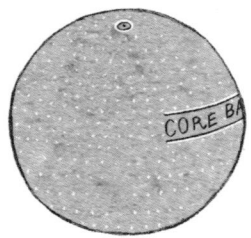

Pilates is a gentle and low-impact form of exercise that often looks deceptively easy – a series of small, slow movements performed with intense concentration. But appearances can be misleading. Done properly, Pilates can be an effective way to build deep core strength, ease chronic back pain and even lift your mood.

What makes Pilates so accessible is its versatility. Whether you're pregnant, recovering from injury, managing arthritis, a top athlete or trying to improve fitness in later life, Pilates offers a safe and effective path to strength. Though often seen as a modern wellness trend, Pilates is over a century old. It was developed by Joseph Pilates, a sickly child born in Germany in 1883, who devoted his life to improving physical health. Young Joseph eventually moved to England, earning a living as a boxer and circus performer before creating a system of movement focused on controlled breathing and precise muscle activation which he called 'Contrology'.

Modern research supports Joseph Pilates' methods. In one trial,[164] just one hour of Pilates per week over 10 weeks significantly boosted strength in sedentary adults. Among athletes, performance improvements have also been recorded: tennis players served faster, and middle-distance runners shaved seconds off their times after regular Pilates practice.

Pilates can also improve mental wellbeing. The emphasis on deep, measured breathing – inhale through the nose, exhale slowly through the mouth – appears to reduce anxiety, promote relaxation and sharpen focus. For many, Pilates serves as much-needed time to reconnect body and mind.

MIND YOUR BACK

One area where evidence of the benefits of Pilates is particularly strong is lower-back pain. In a 2021 randomised controlled trial,[165] people with chronic back pain who took part in an eight-week supervised Pilates programme experienced significantly less pain and improved quality of life compared with those receiving standard care and medication.

Pilates also shows promise for maintaining strength and mobility with age. Professor Ruth Caldeira de Melo of the University of São Paulo has studied its effects for over a decade. In one of her trials,[166] older women took part in mat-based Pilates sessions twice a week for 12 weeks. They showed significant improvements in lower-body strength, dynamic balance and cardiovascular endurance (measuring how far they could walk in six minutes). 'The women who were doing Pilates could walk 30 metres further than they could at the start,' she says.

Another striking finding involved the sit-to-stand test, which is often used by researchers as a reliable predictor of frailty and even longevity. Participants who practised Pilates were found to be able to sit and stand from a chair five times faster, with better control, than those who didn't. 'This matters,' says Melo, 'because better balance and lower-limb strength reduce the risk of falls and help people stay independent for longer.'

She believes the secret benefit of Pilates lies in the way it targets deep stabilising muscles that conventional gym workouts often neglect. 'Pilates looks easy, but it demands well-controlled movements – and full connection between body and mind,' she says.

These benefits haven't gone unnoticed by the world's top athletes. Many professional footballers, runners and tennis players now incorporate Pilates into their training regimens to enhance core strength and flexibility while reducing injury risk. Physiotherapists, in turn, recommend Pilates alongside rehabilitation programmes to rebuild strength and stability in a low-impact way.

For many people, one of the most appealing aspects is how little time you need to get started. 'Even 10 minutes a day can make a difference,' says Melo. She recommends finding a good instructor to help you master the basics. A trained teacher will guide you on breathing techniques and ensure proper alignment, especially if you're dealing with any injuries or chronic conditions. But she says it's also perfectly possible to start at home, with free videos and step-by-step classes available on the NHS website [167] or platforms like YouTube.

What surprises many newcomers is how mentally engaging Pilates can be. Because the movements are subtle, you're encouraged to focus on the tiniest shift of weight or tension. That intense concentration can feel almost meditative. The goal isn't to build bulk or push to exhaustion – it's to retrain your brain and muscles to work together more efficiently. Over time, this re-education translates into improved coordination, a more upright posture and greater ease of movement.

So whether you're recovering from an injury, seeking a calmer mind or simply trying to move with more grace and strength, Pilates might be the surprisingly powerful workout you never knew you needed.

THREE BEGINNER PILATES MOVES TO TRY AT HOME

You don't need fancy equipment to begin reaping the benefits of Pilates. These simple mat-based exercises are ideal for beginners and can be done at home on any soft surface. Focus on slow, controlled movements and steady breathing.

1. THE PELVIC CURL

Lie on your back with your knees bent and feet hip-width apart, your arms by your sides. Inhale to prepare, then exhale as – keeping your knees bent and your feet on the floor – you slowly curl your pelvis to lift your hips and back off the mat, vertebra by vertebra, until your body forms a straight line from shoulders to knees. Inhale at the top, then exhale as you lower with control.

Benefits: Strengthens the glutes, hamstrings and lower back, while improving spinal mobility.

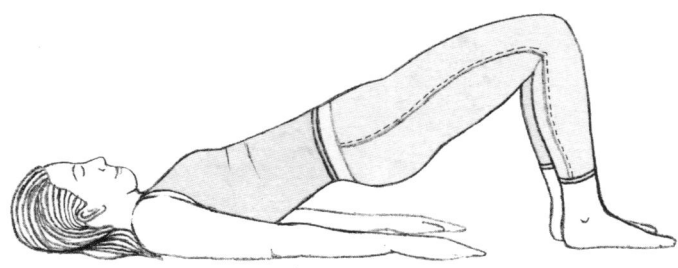

2. THE HUNDRED (MODIFIED)

Lie on your back with your legs in the air, your thighs vertical and your knees bent at 90 degrees. Tuck your chin and lift your head, neck and shoulders off the mat, keeping your tummy pulled in and your back flat to the floor. Extend your arms by your sides, parallel to the floor, and then pulse them up and down while breathing in for five counts and out for five counts. Repeat for 10 breaths.

Benefits: Builds core endurance and teaches breath control.

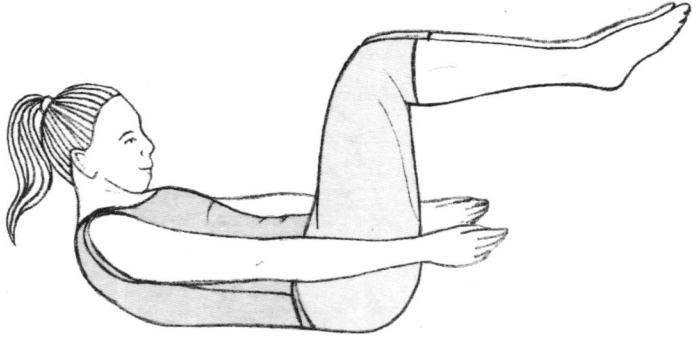

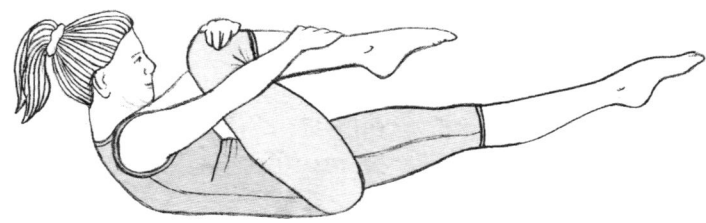

3. SINGLE LEG STRETCH

Lying on your back with head and shoulders lifted from the floor, bring one knee towards your chest while extending the other leg upwards at a 45-degree angle. Switch legs in a scissor-like motion, exhaling with each switch.

Benefits: Engages abdominal muscles and improves coordination and pelvic stability.

just one thing

BE STRONGER AND FITTER

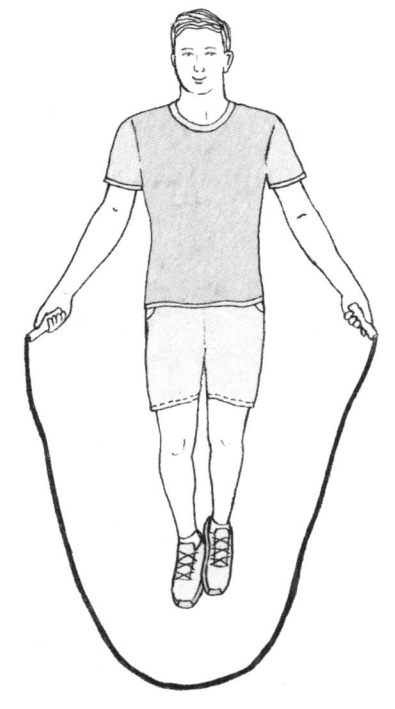

get skipping

How to do it: Skip, jump or hop on one foot for a few minutes each day.

Why do it? It can improve muscle power, bone density and even brain health, including motor control, memory and attention.

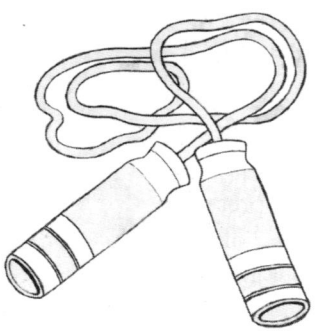

We tend to associate hopping, skipping and jumping with the carefree playtime of childhood, but an emerging body of research suggests these seemingly simple movements could be powerful tools for improving health and longevity in later life. Known collectively as plyometric exercises, the act of hopping or jumping on one or both legs involves explosive movements that encourage rapid stretch and shortening of muscles.

Traditionally the domain of athletes, plyometric training is now being recognised for its potential benefits beyond the sports field. Scientists are discovering that these short, sharp bursts of movement can improve not only physical function but also brain health, bone density and metabolic fitness, particularly in older adults.

The key lies in the way skipping and hopping develops *power* as opposed to strength. While strength allows us to lift heavy things, power (the speed at which a muscle can contract) enables us to react quickly and move with agility. Power is crucial in top-level sport, but it is also incredibly important for the rest of us as we get older if we want to prevent falls, dash for a bus or change direction rapidly without stumbling.

As Professor Urs Granacher from the University of Freiburg, Germany, puts it: 'Power can be described as strength plus speed, and in everyday life, we often need both.'

Unfortunately, muscle power diminishes with age even more quickly than strength does. After the age of 65, muscle power typically declines at a rate of 3 to 4 per cent per year, compared with 1 to 2 per cent for strength. This is because our fast-twitch muscle fibres – the ones that produce short, powerful bursts of movement – are especially vulnerable to the ageing process.

But studies suggest that plyometric exercises such as skipping, hopping and jumping can preserve and even restore some of this power. In a meta-analysis[168] of nine studies on adults aged 50 and over, Professor Granacher and his team found that 12 weeks of jump training – 25 hops, rope skips and squat jumps, three times a week – was enough to significantly improve muscle power.

It might seem easy, but these simple exercises are highly demanding for your neuromuscular system, which is the communication and control network between your brain, nerves and muscles. Every movement we make depends on this system, and our reflexes and balance rely on it working optimally. Professor Granacher's studies show that a little bit of skipping or hopping activates a large number of motor units (these are groups of muscle fibres controlled by a single motor neuron) and forces them to fire rapidly and efficiently. Do it often enough, and this neuromuscular stimulation has been shown to help improve coordination, reaction times and muscular endurance over time.

BUILD STRONG BONES

When you are skipping, hopping or jumping, you land each time with quite a bit of force. This puts a brief but significant load on your bones, which stimulates the formation of bone growth. One study in Hong Kong[169] found that teenage girls who skipped for at least an hour a week had higher bone density than their peers.

More remarkably, a study in women aged 25–50[170] showed that jumping on the spot 20 times, twice a day for 16 weeks, was enough to improve bone mineral density.

Even in post-menopausal women – a group particularly vulnerable to bone weakening and osteoporosis – similar benefits have been reported. In one small study,[171] 20 inactive post-menopausal women were asked to spend three months doing a programme of one-legged jumps every day – on one leg only – and scans showed rapidly improved bone mineral strength in the shin bones of their jumping leg.

BRAIN BOOST

Surprisingly, skipping and hopping can give your brain a boost, too. One study involving students found that rope skipping for 16 minutes three times a week[172] improved short-term memory. Scientists believe the brain boost comes because you are having to synchronise your arms and legs, maintain a rhythm and manage balance. In combination, this challenge works to stimulate brain regions associated with motor control, memory and attention.

'Jumping is a basic, whole-body movement that recruits a wide range of muscle groups and motor units,' explains Granacher. 'The brain has to send signals to fire these muscles in synchrony and at speed. That improves neuromuscular communication.'

For older adults, maintaining this kind of neuromuscular efficiency is critical. Loss of balance, slowed reactions and muscular weakness are all factors that increase your risk of falls and diminish your quality of life as you get older. But jump training, when appropriately scaled, can help address all of these.

For many, even a gentle introduction – hopping on the spot for a few seconds at a time – can bring benefits. As Granacher says: 'You don't need a gym or equipment. You can do these exercises anywhere – even in your living room. And they have a profound effect on your strength, balance, power and health.'

MAKING A SAFE START

Jumping exercises like skipping and hopping may look simple, but if you're unfit, older or prone to joint issues, it's important to build up slowly. Speak to a doctor or physiotherapist before you start if you're concerned, as plyometric movements place considerable force through your joints and muscles. It is essential to start from the right foundation:

1. BUILD BASIC STRENGTH FIRST. Plyometrics are most effective – and safest – when you have a base level of muscle strength, especially in your legs, the core muscles in your abdomen and the glute muscles in your buttocks. Begin with strength-building moves before introducing any jumping. Granacher advises developing a foundation of strength through bodyweight or resistance training (see page 195) before advancing to more explosive movements. Done properly, the risk of injury is low – but overloading the body too soon can lead to problems, he says.

2. FOCUS ON THE LANDING. How you land is more important than how high you jump. Practise 'soft landings' by jumping no more than a few inches off the floor and landing with knees bent, feet hip-width apart, and weight distributed evenly. You should be able to land quietly – noisy landings suggest poor control. Wearing good training shoes with a cushioned midsole will reduce some of the impact of landing.

3. START WITH LOW-IMPACT. Begin with simple movements on a soft surface, such as a carpet or yoga mat. The goal is to build confidence and coordination while gently challenging your body. As fitness improves, you can increase the height of jumps or the duration of each session. Start with short bouts: 10 seconds of jumping followed by 10 seconds of rest, repeated a few times, gradually increasing as your capacity improves.
- ★ **Mini hops:** On a soft surface, hop gently on both feet, then try single-leg hops for 10–15 seconds at a time.
- ★ **Box step-downs:** Step off a low platform (10–15cm high) and practise absorbing the landing.
- ★ **Marching skips:** Lift one knee and do a small jump, alternating sides.

4. KEEP SESSIONS SHORT AND RESTED. Begin with just five minutes of low-impact jumping, hopping or skipping twice a week. Rest between each set. As you build control and endurance, you can gradually increase intensity, volume and complexity – adding in rope skipping or squat jumps.

just one thing

BE STRONGER AND FITTER

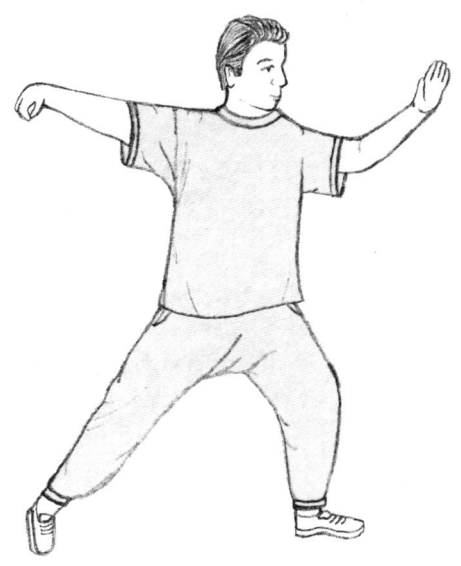

try tai chi

How to do it: Take a tai chi class.

Why do it? It can improve balance, fitness, immunity and mental focus, while lowering the risk of heart disease.

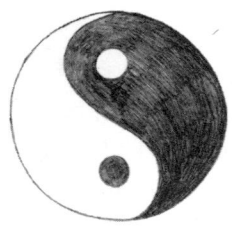

You may have seen videos of older people gathering in parks across China, moving their arms and legs in slow motion. Tai chi might seem like a very gentle form of exercise, but it turns out that the ancient Chinese martial art can not only improve balance but may also benefit your immune system and heart health. Sometimes called shadow boxing and 'meditation in motion', tai chi is, in fact, a series of different postures that are supposed to gently flow into each other in slow movements.

This ancient practice is immensely popular in China. But it is particularly beloved in Hong Kong, where residents have one of the highest life expectancies in the world. Is this connected? Well, possibly. There's certainly a surprising amount of science amassing into the health benefits of tai chi.

One study, for example,[173] which followed 60,000 men in Shanghai for five years, found that those who practise tai chi regularly lived significantly longer than those who didn't. Of course, this could just mean that people who practise tai chi are more careful about other aspects of their health – but perhaps there are other things going on.

Although the movements of tai chi are slow, they do require effort, which raises your heart rate. And crucially, because tai chi is a mix of exercise and meditation, your brain gets a workout as well as your body. In one study[174] that compared tai chi to brisk walking, researchers found that these slow movements were significantly better at reducing not only blood pressure, but also lowering other risk factors for heart disease, such as blood sugar levels and cholesterol.

Not only that, but tai chi could also benefit your immune system. In a fascinating study from the University of California,[175] 100 volunteers were randomly allocated into two groups. Half took tai chi classes for 16 weeks, while the other half took health education classes which included advice on stress, diet and sleep. Both groups received a vaccine against shingles, a painful skin rash which is caused by the same virus as chickenpox. Nine weeks later, the tai chi group showed a more positive immunity response to the vaccine than the control group. They also showed greater improvements in physical functioning, vitality and mental health, and reductions in bodily pain.

And though it looks gentle, it turns out that tai chi can help you lose weight just as effectively as conventional exercise. In fact, it seems to be an excellent way of tackling the visceral fat that can cling to the organs and linger around your tummy.

BRAIN-BOOSTING BONUS

Dr Parco Siu from the University of Hong Kong has been studying the health benefits of tai chi for more than a decade. His research has shown that the gentle movements show benefits for the management of osteoarthritis and for many aspects of cardio, respiratory and musculoskeletal fitness, as well as psychological health.

In one of his studies,[176] his team compared the possible brain-boosting benefits of tai chi with aerobic exercise and muscle-strengthening activities on a group of older adults with mild cognitive impairment. After just three months, the tai chi group started to show improvements in memory and mental flexibility (the ability to switch between tasks), whereas it was six months before the exercise group showed the same kinds of improvements.

'Tai chi seems to work your brain as it works your body,' Dr Siu says. 'Conventional exercise can change the brain a little bit, but not to the extent of what we observe from tai chi training.' In fact, scans show that tai chi can actually increase the density in parts of the brain related to cognitive function and improve connectivity between parts of the brain, indicating it helps the brain to function better. That's why he believes it is important to incorporate the meditative element into the movement practice to make the most of the benefits.

His team also conducted a study looking at tai chi and central obesity,[177] and found tai chi to be just as effective as aerobic exercise and muscle-strengthening activities for reducing waist circumference and central obesity. 'If you look at the people who practise tai chi, it doesn't look as if they're exercising,' he says. 'But people practising tai chi burn a similar number of calories compared to conventional exercise.' This is really good news for people who struggle to exercise or who prefer not to.

So why not give tai chi a try? You'll find videos on the BBC website[178] and also on YouTube. Aim to practise for 15 minutes a day, every day. If you like it, Dr Siu recommends finding a class supervised by a qualified instructor. 'The bodily movements are not difficult to pick up from watching videos online, but the meditation is more difficult,' he explains. 'The effect is more powerful if someone can guide you and lead you in the moving meditation to maximise the benefits – and the enjoyment!'

TAI CHI EXERCISES

1. COMMENCEMENT
- Stand with your feet shoulder-width apart, knees slightly bent, and arms relaxed by your sides.
- Inhale slowly through your nose as you raise both arms in front of you to shoulder height, palms facing down.
- Exhale through your mouth as you gently lower your arms.
- Focus on coordinating breath and movement. Repeat 3–5 times.

Benefits: This introductory movement calms the mind, promotes proper posture and introduces breath control.

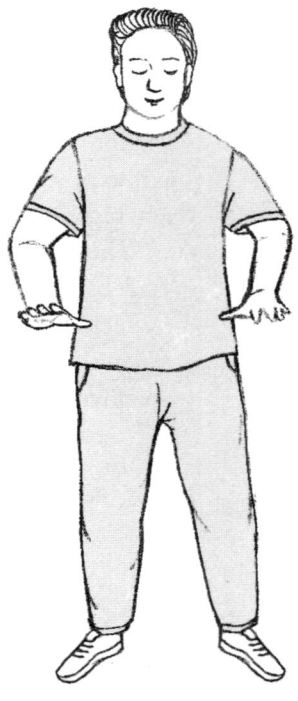

2. PARTING THE WILD HORSE'S MANE

· From standing, step one foot forwards and shift your weight onto it.
· As you step, move one hand forwards and slightly to the side (as if stroking a horse), while the other hand sweeps back and down by your hip.
· Alternate sides slowly with each step.

Benefits: This exercise improves coordination and balance.

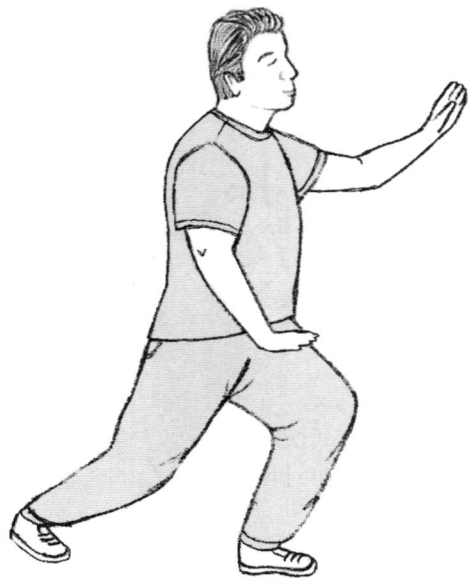

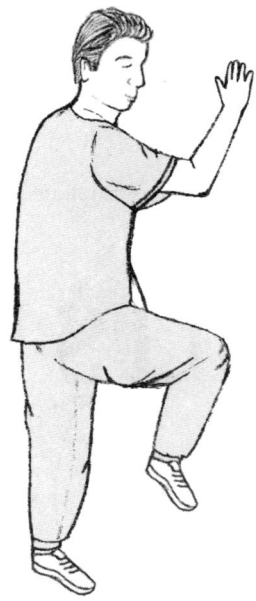

3. GOLDEN ROOSTER STANDS ON ONE LEG

- Stand tall with your feet shoulder-width apart, knees soft, and arms relaxed by your sides.
- Shift your weight slowly onto your left leg, grounding through your foot.
- As you inhale, lift your right knee gently in front of you to about hip height (or as high as feels stable).
- At the same time, raise your left hand (opposite hand to leg) to chest height, palm facing forwards as if to 'block', and bring your right hand down beside your right hip, palm facing in, like you're gently pressing downwards.
- Hold for a breath, then slowly lower your leg and arms.
- Repeat on the other side.

Benefits: This challenges your balance and strengthens your legs, ankles and core, improving single-leg stability and enhancing mental focus.

just
one
thing

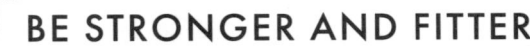

BE STRONGER AND FITTER

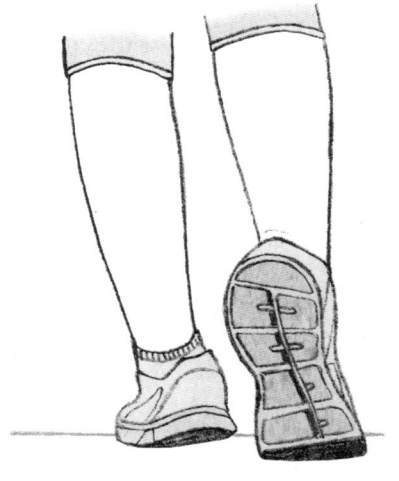

walk backwards

How to do it: Build a few minutes of backwards walking into your exercise regime.

Why do it? This can improve stability and balance, ease lower back pain and boost memory and brain power.

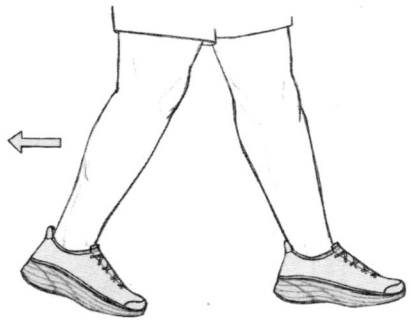

Backwards walking – or retro walking as it's sometimes known – isn't just a quirky fitness trend. It's a low-impact activity with deep roots, stretching back to traditional Chinese medicine, where the saying goes: 'A hundred steps backwards are worth a thousand steps forwards.' It might look a bit eccentric, but the simple act of walking backwards is an excellent way to improve both your balance and your brain function.

One of the early American pioneers was Patrick Harman, who more than a century ago walked backwards from San Francisco to New York City. More recently, backwards walking has been taken up by physiotherapists as a treatment for back pain, balance and gait. Now, studies are showing that walking backwards could also ease lower back pain and even boost your memory.

A FITNESS CHALLENGE
The first thing to know is that walking backwards is harder than walking forwards – in a good way. According to a small study from the University of Stellenbosch in South Africa,[179] backwards walking

burns around 30 per cent more energy than forwards walking at the same pace. Volunteers in the study who added retro walking to their weekly routine lost an average of 2.5 per cent of their body fat – without any change to their diet.

That's because, when we walk backwards, we use muscles that are usually underworked: the calves and shins, and the quadriceps at the front of the thigh, get far more engagement. A Texan study[180] found that blood lactate levels – which are an indicator of muscular effort – were three times higher during backwards walking than ordinary walking.

Despite the effort required, it is good to know that backwards walking is much more gentle on the knees and back. Professor Janet Dufek, from the University of Nevada, Las Vegas, who has been studying backwards walking for over 30 years, explains: 'When you walk forwards, you land on the heel and push off with the forefoot, but in backwards walking, you tend to land on the ball of the foot and very often the heel doesn't even touch the ground.' This subtle shift results in a lower impact on joints. 'To walk backwards safely, you need to engage your core muscles, pull back your shoulders and lift your chest,' says Professor Dufek. That alone may help ease the load on the spine.

Although clearly a fan, she claims to have been surprised by how effective backwards walking seems to be for improving flexibility and reducing back pain. In one of her studies,[181] a small group of athletes with recurring back twinges added five weeks of backwards walking to their routine, and over 80 per cent of them reported a reduction in their back pain. Another small study[182] tracked older adults who were asked to walk backwards for 15 minutes a day, four times a week. By the end of four weeks, participants had greater flexibility and reduced stiffness in the lumbar (lower) spine.

One contributing factor is thought to be the hamstrings – the muscles at the back of the thigh – which can become tight if you sit for prolonged periods. Backwards walking gently stretches these muscles, improving the range of motion in your hips and helping to rebalance the pelvis and lower back.

IT'S ALL IN THE HEAD

What's perhaps more surprising is the effect of walking backwards on the brain. In a study by researchers at the University of Roehampton,[183] volunteers were asked to watch a short video and then either walk forwards, walk backwards, or stand still. When later tested on their memory of what they'd seen on the video, the backwards walkers' recall ability consistently outperformed those who walked normally.

The theory is that because reverse walking is an unfamiliar gait, it places unusual demands on the brain, forcing it to recruit more executive function. The prefrontal cortex – the part responsible for planning, problem-solving and decision-making – lights up when we walk backwards. In other words, doing something out of the ordinary like this activates important parts of the brain.

Another small study[184] found that people who walked backwards had faster reaction times – a sign of enhanced neural processing. While the precise mechanism isn't fully understood, there's a growing belief that challenging the brain in new ways (especially in combination with movement) could even help delay age-related cognitive decline.

FINDING BALANCE

Perhaps the most immediate benefit of backwards walking is improved balance. Because backwards walking removes visual cues – you can't see where you're going – it forces your body to rely more heavily on the vestibular (inner ear) and proprioceptive (muscle and joint awareness) systems.

In one of Professor Dufek's trials,[185] elderly volunteers who practised backwards walking for 15 minutes a day on a treadmill for four weeks showed significant improvements in stability. This, she says, makes it a useful exercise in fall prevention.

So how do you begin – without bumping into trees or parked cars? Start slowly, says Dufek. 'Try one or two minutes at a time and add an extra minute every couple of days.' The aim is to build to five minutes of backwards walking, five days a week.

'You'll know it's working when you start to feel different muscles engage,' says Dufek. 'And you'll likely notice improvements in your posture, too.' It may look eccentric, but retro walking is oddly soothing once you find your rhythm. You can feel the different muscle groups firing, your core stabilising, and – after a few sessions – perhaps even your brain ticking a little faster, too.

TIPS FOR BACKWARDS WALKING

1. DO IT WITH A FRIEND. If retro walking outdoors, go with a friend who can spot for you while you're getting started, which is especially useful in avoiding unexpected obstacles. Face each other, hold hands and take turns walking backwards while the other walks forwards as a guide.

2. START SLOWLY AND ON FLAT GROUND. Begin with short sessions (2–5 minutes) on a flat, familiar, open surface. The safest place to begin is a hallway, park path or gym corridor. You can walk along a corridor with your fingers tracing a wall beside you for light support. This helps you get used to the unfamiliar movement pattern without risking tripping or falling.

3. USE A MIRROR. If you have access to a gym studio, practise walking backwards in front of the mirror.

4. USE A TREADMILL. Many people find walking backwards on a treadmill helpful because you can hold on to the side rails for balance.

5. FOCUS ON POSTURE AND CORE ENGAGEMENT. Stand tall, keep your shoulders back, and engage your core. Look over your shoulder periodically to check your path but avoid craning your neck the entire time. Controlled posture helps prevent strain and improves coordination.

6. ADD VARIETY GRADUALLY. Once you're confident walking backwards on the flat, try light inclines. Backwards walking uphill can engage different muscle groups, including your glutes and calves. Alternate between walking forwards and backwards in intervals.

just
one
thing

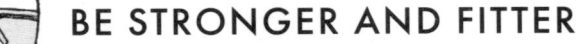

BE STRONGER AND FITTER

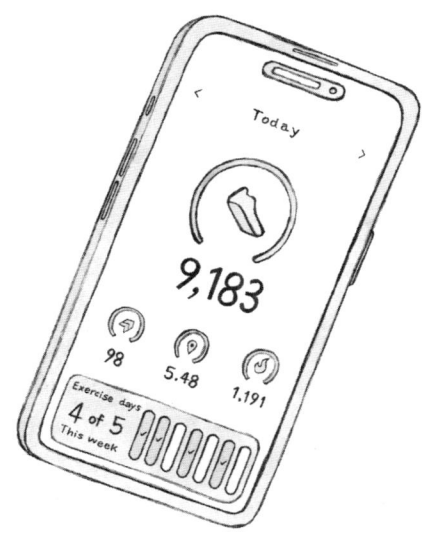

track your
exercise

How to do it: Use a tracking device to monitor your activity levels.

Why do it? It can help to improve fitness, heart health, mood and brain function.

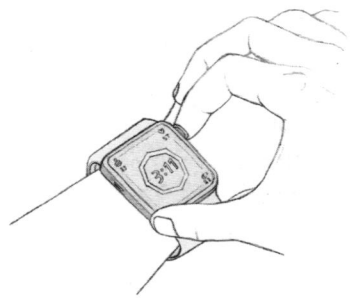

We all know that being active is incredibly good for our health, but despite our best intentions, few of us consistently hit the recommended guidelines of 150 minutes of moderate-intensity activity a week. Now, a growing body of fascinating research shows that you're significantly more likely to move if you use some form of technology to track your steps. This is important, because there is no doubt that increasing your activity levels can make a profound difference to your mental and physical wellbeing.

The idea that we must aim for 10,000 steps a day has become ingrained, but it is also intimidating. But encouragingly, a recent meta-analysis involving more than 220,000 participants[186] found that walking just 4,000 steps a day is enough to start reducing your risk of dying prematurely from any natural cause. The benefits were consistent across all age groups. Some movement, it seems, is good. But more is always better. In fact, every additional 1,000 steps taken beyond that baseline is linked to a 15 per cent reduction in the risk of early death.

And, importantly, you stand a much better chance of reaching and sticking at those healthy targets if you use some sort of technology to track your activity progress. Using a wearable fitness tracker, or even just logging your daily step count on your smartphone, has been shown to be a great way to keep you accountable – if you check in regularly, it can be like having a personal trainer in your pocket, urging you to keep up the good work.

The good news is that you don't necessarily need to spend money on a high-end fitness tracker to access these benefits. Fitness tracking has evolved into a booming global industry, and around one-third of UK adults own a smartwatch or fitness band. But approximately 90 per cent of UK adults own a smartphone, and the majority of these come with built-in health-monitoring features.

Professor Carol Maher, an expert in digital health and physical activity at the University of South Australia, has spent years studying the effects of fitness trackers. 'Anything that helps you track your activity and become more aware of your daily movement is valuable,' she says. 'Smartphone apps are great for this: they count your steps and allow you to monitor progress over time. But the main downside is that, unless you carry your phone in your pocket at all times, you may miss a fair proportion of your steps.'

When it comes to measuring the intensity of movement, many experts agree that fitness wearables tend to offer more precision. These devices provide detailed graphs and combine various data points to estimate active minutes, heart rate and even sleep quality.

THE CRUCIAL SIX EXTRA MINUTES
Maher and her team analysed data from 39 systematic reviews, which collectively gathered performance data from over 163,000 participants.[187] They concluded that wearable activity trackers are consistently associated with increased levels of physical activity. On average, people who used trackers walked an additional 1,800 steps per day, added 14 minutes of walking to their daily routine, and performed around six extra minutes of moderate to vigorous physical activity – compared to those who didn't track their activity levels at all.

'That might not sound like much,' Maher says, 'but even adding 5–10 minutes of physical activity a day has measurable benefits for heart health, metabolic function and mental wellbeing. The six minutes of extra vigorous activity is where the real magic happens.'

That's because six minutes of vigorous activity has been shown to have a big impact on your mental functioning. In one study conducted by researchers at University College London,[188] more than 4,000 middle-aged adults wore activity monitors. The participants who performed just six minutes more of moderate to vigorous exercise each day showed better cognitive performance, including sharper memory and faster processing speeds, than those who skipped the extra six minutes.

Maher argues that even small, incremental gains are worthwhile. 'Wearables provide a real motivational boost. They encourage people to become active participants in their health journey,' she says. Sceptics might suggest that those who buy activity trackers are already inclined to be more active, which could be skewing the results. But Maher and her colleagues have conducted rigorous randomised controlled trials to tease apart cause and effect.

In one study,[189] participants were randomly assigned either a very basic tracker that collected data, sending it directly to the lab with no feedback to the user, or a consumer-grade tracker with real-time feedback, goal-setting features, plus prompts to get up and move if the user had been sitting for too long. 'The only difference between the two groups was the interactivity of the device,' she explains. And the result? 'The group with feedback consistently moved more.'

So what's going on? 'Wearables help people understand their current activity level, set meaningful goals and monitor progress. These psychological and behavioural tools are incredibly powerful,' Maher explains. 'They effectively give people a sense of agency over their own health.'

Ultimately, the goal isn't perfection. It's progress. And the growing consensus is that even modest daily increases in movement can yield surprisingly large benefits for longevity, heart health, mood and brain function. If a wearable device can help you make those changes, it might be a simple investment that is well worth making.

MAKE THE MOST OUT OF YOUR TRACKING DEVICE

1. FIGURE OUT YOUR DEVICE. Take time to work out the full functionality of your device – don't just switch it on and hope for the best! Watch any instructional videos offered.

2. TRACK MODERATE-TO-VIGOROUS ACTIVITY TIME. Set your device to track only brisk walking, cycling or swimming – rather than just step counts.

3. CHECK YOUR TRACKER REGULARLY. Don't just check before bed at night: always check at midday and adjust accordingly. Think of it as a coach on your wrist.

4. USE THE DATA TO PLAN AHEAD. If it's 3pm and you're well below your target, plan an evening walk or a vigorous activity.

5. ENABLE 'MOVE' REMINDERS. Treat these hourly prompts to stand or walk as non-negotiable mini-breaks. Even 1–2 minutes of movement when you've been sitting for a while can improve blood sugar control and circulation.

6. JOIN STEP OR ACTIVITY CHALLENGES. Join with friends or colleagues, as social accountability can increase activity by up to 30 per cent.

7. COMPETE AGAINST YOURSELF. Try to beat your own best days or weeks to build a 'streak' habit.

8. SET WEEKLY OR MONTHLY GOALS. Reward yourself when you hit them.

just one thing

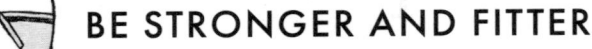

BE STRONGER AND FITTER

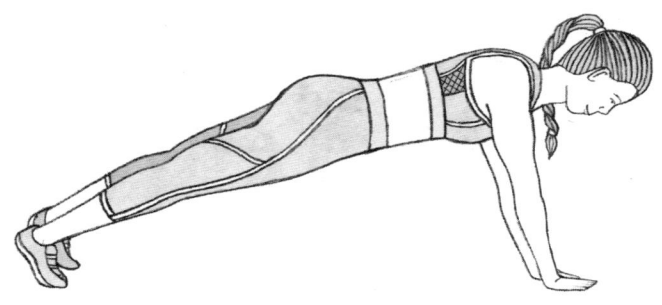

do planks

How to do it: Hold a plank position every day.

Why do it? Doing planks can improve strength, balance, coordination, posture and blood pressure.

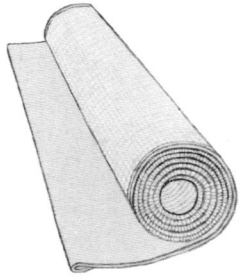

The plank is a very simple exercise where you hold your body in a rigid straight line with only your hands or forearms and toes touching the floor. It might look easy, but maintaining that rigid hold for seconds, even minutes, requires quite a bit of strength, and considering the fact that you're not actually moving at all, it is a surprisingly effective way to build strength and improve balance, coordination and posture. There's also fascinating research to show that static holds like this are an effective way to lower blood pressure.

When you're trying to maintain a straight line from shoulder to toes in a plank, or sitting on an imaginary chair against the wall (the 'wall sit') for upwards of 30 seconds, you will be doing what exercise physiologists call 'isometric exercises'. The term comes from the Greek '*iso*' (same) and '*metron*' (measure), meaning that the muscle holds its length: you are activating important muscles without actually lengthening or shortening them.

Isometric exercises look very simple, but the physiological ripple effects of keeping your body completely still under tension are powerful. It turns out that the effort it takes to resist gravity and maintain a perfect wall squat or plank activates deep stabilising muscles in the lower back and core that support your spine and pelvis – muscles that are notoriously hard to reach with more conventional movements. There is exciting new research to show that isometric exercises can help to lower your blood pressure more effectively than other, more conventional types of exercise. When scientists from Penn State University in the USA attached electrodes to 20 participants[190] while they did core exercises to measure how hard their muscles worked, they concluded that holding a plank works your core muscles a lot harder than doing traditional abdominal exercises such as crunches or oblique twists.

Researchers think that's because planks don't just target the 'six-pack' muscles on the front of your abdomen; they engage other muscles, including your obliques (which run along the sides of your torso), back extensors (which flank the spine), glutes (the buttocks), shoulders and even your hip flexors at the front of your pelvis. This three-dimensional engagement builds a much more functional core, which is important not just for athletes but for anyone hoping to avoid the hunched posture, stiff joints and niggling backaches of modern life. A strong core means fewer injuries, better posture and balance, and perhaps most importantly, less back pain, which is one of the leading causes of disability worldwide.

In one small study,[191] 30 young men and women with lower-back pain did a few minutes of daily plank exercises, including the side plank, where you lean on one arm. Each exercise was held for only 20 to 30 seconds. After just three weeks, they reported significantly less pain and a bigger improvement in their quality of life.

A FIX FOR HIGH BLOOD PRESSURE

Perhaps more surprisingly, isometric exercises may be one of the most effective forms of exercise for lowering blood pressure, too. Dr Jamie O'Driscoll, a cardiovascular physiologist at Canterbury Christ Church University in Kent, became interested in the phenomenon after observing earlier studies on pilots, where simple handgrip exercises – squeezing a tennis-ball-sized gauge – had unexpectedly led to lower blood pressure readings.

It seemed improbable that exercising such a small muscle group could produce such significant cardiovascular effects, so Dr O'Driscoll began to investigate more systematically. In one of his trials,[192] he and his team studied older adults with mild to moderate hypertension (high blood pressure). Participants performed isometric exercises such as planks and wall squats daily for four weeks. Each session lasted only a few minutes, yet the results were impressive: participants saw a substantial drop in blood pressure.

To dig deeper, Dr O'Driscoll led a 2023 meta-analysis[193] comparing over 270 exercise trials, which included all major forms of physical activity, from traditional aerobic training to resistance training, high-intensity interval training (HIIT) and isometric holds. The analysis revealed that isometric exercise produced the largest average reduction in blood pressure and outperformed even brisk walking and HIIT.

He believes this is caused by the way isometric holds force your blood vessels to contract for an extended time. When you hold a squat or a plank, the contracting muscles temporarily restrict blood flow. But when the hold ends, blood rushes back through the arteries. This 'reperfusion' effect causes the lining of the arteries (the endothelium) to release nitric oxide, a molecule that helps blood vessels widen and become more flexible. Do a plank often enough, and this improved vascular flexibility means your arteries become better able to accommodate the natural fluctuations in blood flow that occur throughout the day, which in turn helps to lower your overall blood pressure.

Isometric training also appears to stimulate the parasympathetic nervous system – the branch responsible for rest and recovery – while dampening the 'fight or flight' response of the sympathetic nervous system. Over time, this can lead to lower resting heart rate and blood pressure, as well as improved cardiovascular health. Dr O'Driscoll explains that these benefits are long-lasting: 'We're seeing real, long-term changes in how blood vessels behave, especially in people with high blood pressure,' he says.

One big advantage of planks and wall sits is you don't need a gym or a personal trainer to benefit from these exercises, and they are achievable for people who may find other forms of exercise difficult. If you have joint issues, are recovering from injury or are new to fitness, they can offer a low-impact, time-efficient option that still delivers significant results.

If you do have hypertension, check with your doctor before beginning a new exercise programme. But for most people, a short daily routine of planks and wall sits could be a simple and surprisingly powerful intervention.

HOW TO WALL SIT

Stand with your back against a strong, stable wall and take a step out. Now slowly slide your bottom down that wall so your knees are bent. Start with a small bend in the knee, but as your strength improves and this becomes easier, progress to having your knees at right angles, with your thighs parallel to the floor. Hold for 30 seconds, rest and repeat four times, increasing the duration of the hold as you get stronger.

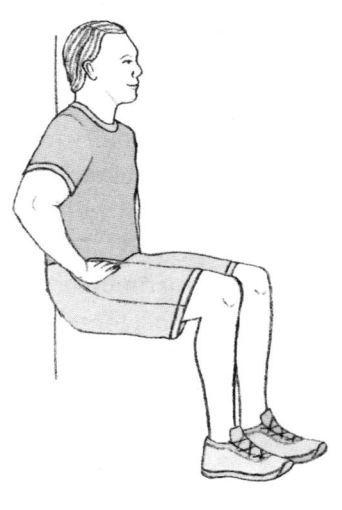

HOW TO PLANK

1. WORKING UP TO THE PLANK

Complete beginners can try these steps:

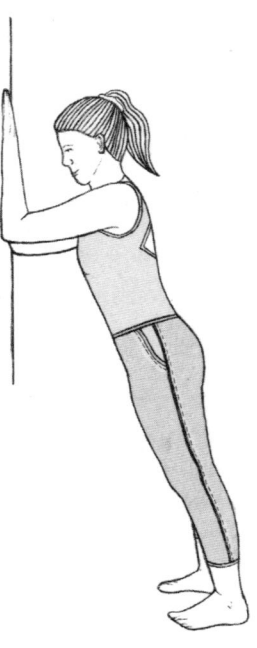

* Start by facing a wall, standing arms-length away with your feet hip-width apart.

  Place your palms flat on the wall at shoulder height, shoulder-width apart, fingers pointing upwards.

* Walk your feet back a little, keeping your body in a straight line from head to heels, aiming for a 45-degree angle.

* Tuck in your ribs, pull in your tummy (to activate your core muscles), squeeze your buttock muscles (glutes) and breathe steadily.

* Hold for 10–30 seconds, then slowly walk your feet forwards and lower your hands from the wall.

* When this becomes easy, progress to holding a plank with your hands on a countertop or table, stepping back so your body is in a straight line from head to heels.

* When this becomes easy, progress to planking on all-fours on the floor. Bring your forearms to the floor under your shoulders and step your knees backwards so your body from head to knees is a straight line.

* When this becomes easy, progress to the full plank.

2. THE FULL PLANK

Lie face down with your forearms on the floor, your legs extended and your feet together. Push into your forearms as you raise your body so it forms a straight line from your head and your neck to your feet. Your weight should be on your forearms and the balls of your feet. Make sure your back stays straight. Try to engage your abdominal muscles. Hold for 30 seconds or more. Rest, then repeat four times.

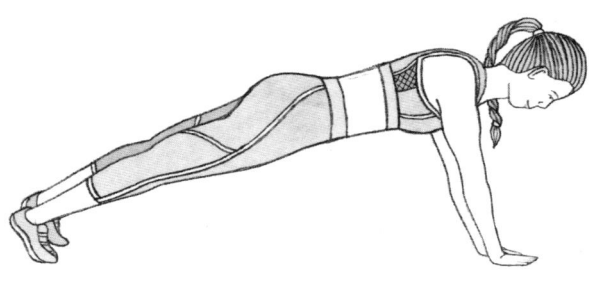

3. WORKING UP TO THE SIDE PLANK

Beginners can try these steps:

⭑ Lie on your side with knees bent at 90 degrees, stacking your knees and feet together.

⭑ Place your bottom forearm on the floor, elbow directly under your shoulder.

⭑ Engage your core and glutes, then press your forearm into the floor and lift your hips until your body forms a straight line from knees to head. Hold for 20–60 seconds.

⭑ Gently bring your hips back to the floor and switch sides.

When this becomes easy, progress to straightening the top leg only, keeping the bottom leg bent for support.

⭑ When this becomes easy, try the full side plank but with feet staggered – one slightly in front of the other to increase your stability.

4. THE FULL SIDE PLANK

Lie on your side with your legs extended and stacked one on top of the other. Prop yourself up on your bottom forearm so your elbow is directly under your shoulder. Engage your core and lift your hips off the floor, forming a straight line from your shoulders to your feet. Your top hand can rest on your hip or be extended to the ceiling for added challenge. Hold this position for 15–30 seconds to start. Focus on keeping your hips lifted and your body aligned – don't let yourself tip forwards or backwards. Switch sides.

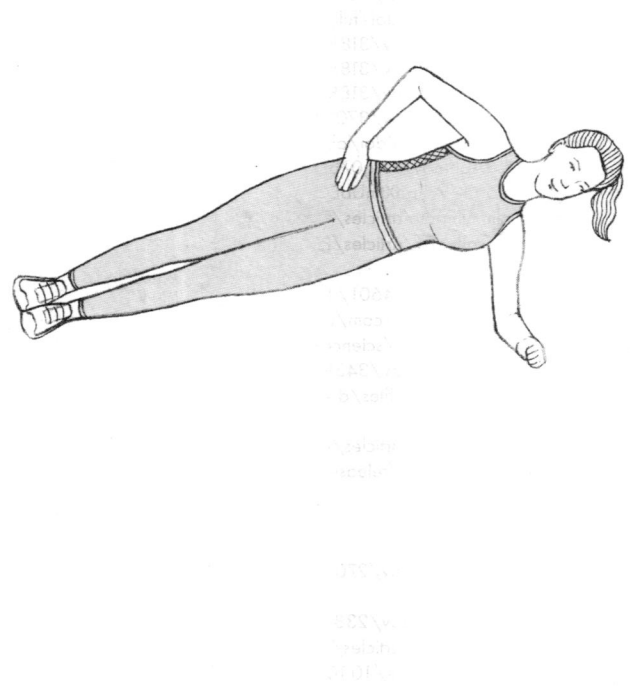

Endnotes

Introduction

1   https://onlinelibrary.wiley.com/doi/epdf/10.1002/ejsp.674

Boost your mood

2   https://www.mdpi.com/2072-6643/14/6/1189
3   https://pmc.ncbi.nlm.nih.gov/articles/PMC7352411/#:~:text=Those%20in%20the%20
     curcumin%20group%20had%20significantly,needs%20to%20be%20replicated%20
     with%20larger%20numbers
4   https://pmc.ncbi.nlm.nih.gov/articles/PMC8590273/
5   https://pubmed.ncbi.nlm.nih.gov/36610110
6   https://pmc.ncbi.nlm.nih.gov/articles/PMC7446227/#Sec10
7   https://researchgate.net/publication/359084051_PM25_decrease_with_
     precipitation_as_revealed_by_single-point_ground-based_observation
8   https://pmc.ncbi.nlm.nih.gov/articles/PMC9564959/
9   https://www.library.hbs.edu/working-knowledge/blue-skies-distractions-arise-how-
     weather-affects-productivity
10   https://psychiatryonline.org/doi/10.1176/pn.42.1.0025
11   https://www.tandfonline.com/doi/full/10.1080/17439760.2022.2154695
12   https://pubmed.ncbi.nlm.nih.gov/31888986
13   https://pubmed.ncbi.nlm.nih.gov/31888986
14   https://pubmed.ncbi.nlm.nih.gov/31888986
15   https://pubmed.ncbi.nlm.nih.gov/37036113/
16   https://onlinelibrary.wiley.com/doi/abs/10.1111/psyp.12578?casa_token=O59K
     x4piQVwAAAAA%3AgNnqy2KHg07bZCq1msgGJT24Y-giB_Cd5A_FWe8147I_
     foJUcwHOtt5sMnZ6o2--WZpoXtmUbECHRw
17   https://pmc.ncbi.nlm.nih.gov/articles/PMC10752423/
18   https://pmc.ncbi.nlm.nih.gov/articles/PMC6427672/#:~:text=5.,of%20diseases%20
     and/or%20disabilities.
19   https://www.mdpi.com/1660-4601/19/21/13874
20   https://www.medicalnewstoday.com/articles/66840#1
21   https://www.sciencedirect.com/science/article/abs/pii/S0048969719346753
22   https://pubmed.ncbi.nlm.nih.gov/34388212/
23   https://lluh.org/sites/lluh.org/files/docs/LIVE-IT-Bain-Article-Effect-of-Humor-Whole-
     Person.pdf
24   https://pmc.ncbi.nlm.nih.gov/articles/PMC5037252/
25   https://www.sciencedaily.com/releases/2005/03/050309111444.htm

Support brain health

26   https://pubmed.ncbi.nlm.nih.gov/27083496/; https://pmc.ncbi.nlm.nih.gov/articles/
     PMC6316673/
27   https://pubmed.ncbi.nlm.nih.gov/23866098/
28   https://pmc.ncbi.nlm.nih.gov/articles/PMC8127249/
29   https://link.springer.com/article/10.1007/s00394-017-1513-0
30   https://www.researchgate.net/publication/352942510_Abstract_5132_Positive_
     Emotions_and_the_Endothelium_Does_Joyful_Music_Improve_Vascular_Health

31   https://www.news-medical.net/news/20241018/Music-aids-recovery-after-surgery.aspx

32   https://medicine.cnsu.edu/news/PDFs/2024-10-18-Listening_to_music_may_speed_up_recovery.pdf

33   https://www.tandfonline.com/eprint/eJz5eH7qiMmZCePXHWpE/full

34   https://www.sciencedaily.com/releases/2008/10/081001093753.htm

35   https://kb.osu.edu/server/api/core/bitstreams/6d6496e5-b378-4bc1-94d9-da63f3204001/content

36   https://pmc.ncbi.nlm.nih.gov/articles/PMC4790847/

37   https://www.nature.com/articles/s41598-022-23340-4

38   https://www.researchgate.net/publication/358459375_Piano_Training_Enhances_Executive_Functions_and_Psychosocial_Outcomes_in_Aging_Results_of_a_Randomized_Controlled_Trial

39   https://www.researchgate.net/publication/258337304_Effects_of_music_learning_and_piano_practice_on_cognitive_function_mood_and_quality_of_life_in_older_adults

40   https://www.bmj.com/content/340/bmj.c2451

41   https://pmc.ncbi.nlm.nih.gov/articles/PMC11657933/

42   https://pubmed.ncbi.nlm.nih.gov/35946825/

43   https://www.ahajournals.org/doi/full/10.1161/JAHA.119.012330

44   https://www.sciencedirect.com/science/article/pii/S266724212400112X

45   https://aap.onlinelibrary.wiley.com/doi/abs/10.1002/JPER.17-0149

46   https://www.cochrane.org/evidence/CD002281_poweredelectric-toothbrushes-compared-manual-toothbrushes-maintaining-oral-health

47   https://onlinelibrary.wiley.com/doi/full/10.1111/idj.12571?utm_source=chatgpt.com

48   https://onlinelibrary.wiley.com/doi/pdf/10.1111/ipd.13130

49   https://pubmed.ncbi.nlm.nih.gov/31743654/

50   https://www.sciencedaily.com/releases/2018/05/180531190840.htm

51   https://pubmed.ncbi.nlm.nih.gov/18326618/

52   https://pubmed.ncbi.nlm.nih.gov/33042566/

53   https://pubmed.ncbi.nlm.nih.gov/25714035/#:~:text=Discussion:%20Our%20findings%20provide%20further%20evidence%20for,in%20cognitive%20function%2C%20specifically%20alertness%20and%20attention.

54   https://pubmed.ncbi.nlm.nih.gov/35816192/

55   https://www.neurology.org/doi/10.1212/WNL.0000000000000755

56   https://www.medrxiv.org/content/10.1101/2024.11.21.24317708v1.full

57   https://www.researchgate.net/publication/377801361_The_associations_of_serum_vitamin_D_status_and_vitamin_D_supplements_use_with_all-cause_dementia_Alzheimer's_disease_and_vascular_dementia_a_UK_Biobank_based_prospective_cohort_study

58   https://www.nmn.com/news/daily-vitamin-d-supplementation-slows-cellular-aging-new-trial-finds

59   https://pmc.ncbi.nlm.nih.gov/articles/PMC8228257/#:~:text=The%20results%20showed%20more%20brain%20activation%20and,cerebellum%2C%20left%20and%20right%20inferior%20parietal%20gyrus.

60   https://www.nature.com/articles/s41562-019-0556-z

61   https://pubmed.ncbi.nlm.nih.gov/8971255/

62   https://www.consciousbreathing.com/blogs/co2-academy/humming-can-eliminate-sinusitis?srsltid=AfmBOoqt5_C2ynyMXGGk_KmsjpagjEptvHGpwX1KKR89x1ZUbEe6846h

Reduce stress

63 https://explodingtopics.com/blog/smartphone-usage-stats
64 https://www.journals.uchicago.edu/doi/full/10.1086/691462
https://news.utexas.edu/2017/06/26/the-mere-presence-of-your-smartphone-reduces-brain-power/
65 https://guilfordjournals.com/doi/10.1521/jscp.2018.37.10.751
66 https://link.springer.com/article/10.1007/s41347-023-00304-7
67 https://pubmed.ncbi.nlm.nih.gov/26957754/
68 https://pubmed.ncbi.nlm.nih.gov/25393825/
69 https://www.sciencedirect.com/science/article/pii/S0003687016301235
70 https://www.ncbi.nlm.nih.gov/pmc/articles/PMC7320888/
71 https://psycnet.apa.org/doiLanding?doi=10.1037%2Fxap0000430
72 https://web.archive.org/web/20160304110701/http://homepage.psy.utexas.edu/HomePage/Faculty/Pennebaker/Reprints/Beall1986.pdf
73 https://psycnet.apa.org/doiLanding?doi=10.1037%2F0022-006X.63.5.787
74 https://pmc.ncbi.nlm.nih.gov/articles/PMC1150330/#:~:text=The%20results%20showed%20that%20the,different%20types%20of%20surgery.%22%20%E2%80%A6
75 https://pubmed.ncbi.nlm.nih.gov/12377959/
76 Pennebaker, J W, & Smyth, J M, *Opening Up by Writing It Down: How Expressive Writing Improves Health and Eases Emotional Pain*, Guilford Press, New York, 2016; https://www.researchgate.net/publication/6845771_Benefits_of_Expressive_Writing_in_Lowering_Rumination_and_Depressive_Symptoms
77 https://pubmed.ncbi.nlm.nih.gov/28056735/
78 https://link.springer.com/article/10.1007/s00213-006-0573-2
79 https://ajcn.nutrition.org/article/S0002-9165(23)13551-9/fulltext
80 https://pubmed.ncbi.nlm.nih.gov/36037472/
81 https://pubmed.ncbi.nlm.nih.gov/33622762/
82 https://www.liebertpub.com/doi/10.1089/jpm.2015.0528
83 https://www.tandfonline.com/doi/full/10.1080/08893675.2023.2250921
84 https://www.researchgate.net/publication/11273302_Effects_of_speech_therapy_with_poetry_on_heart_rate_rhythmicity_and_cardiorespiratory_coordination
85 https://www.researchgate.net/profile/Malvina-Garner/publication/331689520_10-Week_Hatha_Yoga_Increases_Right_Hippocampal_Density_Compared_to_Active_and_Passive_Control_Groups_A_Controlled_Structural_cMRI_Study/links/5ee686b1299bf1faac55dc83/10-Week-Hatha-Yoga-Increases-Right-Hippocampal-Density-Compared-to-Active-and-Passive-Control-Groups-A-Controlled-Structural-cMRI-Study.pdf
86 https://www.medscape.com/viewarticle/880975#vp_2
87 https://www.researchgate.net/publication/377105859_Yoga_unraveling_the_internal_pharmacy_-_Impact_on_genome_and_epigenome
88 https://pubmed.ncbi.nlm.nih.gov/32982898/

Manage your weight

89 https://www.kcl.ac.uk/news/quarter-people-unhealthy-snacking
90 https://www.bmj.com/content/385/bmj-2023-078476
91 https://pmc.ncbi.nlm.nih.gov/articles/PMC9899573/
92 https://www.kcl.ac.uk/news/late-night-snacks-unfavourable-health
93 https://westminsterresearch.westminster.ac.uk/download/1b3e2e484825641d-9a62d0ed0a012f7c6405a35b48e7db2929ef39c8856bd2e2/895010/nqaa100.pdf

94   https://www.sciencedaily.com/releases/2021/05/210528114107.htm#:~:text=A%20
genetic%20study%20of%20840%2C000,in%20the%20journal%20JAMA%20Psychiatry
95   https://www.bu.edu/articles/2019/cerebrospinal-fluid-washing-in-brain-during-sleep/
96   https://academic.oup.com/ehjdh/article/2/4/658/6423198?login=false
97   https://jamanetwork.com/journals/jamainternalmedicine/fullarticle/2788694
98   https://business.yougov.com/content/51613-how-people-in-the-uk-prefer-to-cook-from-
scratch-or-meal-kits
99   https://www.bmj.com/content/384/bmj-2023-077310
100 https://ijbnpa.biomedcentral.com/articles/10.1186/s12966-017-0567-y
101 https://www.cell.com/cell-metabolism/fulltext/S1550-4131(19)30248-7
102 https://dom-pubs.onlinelibrary.wiley.com/doi/10.1111/dom.15922 ; https://pmc.ncbi.
nlm.nih.gov/articles/PMC8532572/
103 https://pmc.ncbi.nlm.nih.gov/articles/PMC6357517/
104 https://pubmed.ncbi.nlm.nih.gov/32927895/
105 https://pmc.ncbi.nlm.nih.gov/articles/PMC6356451/#:~:text=Cardiovascular%20
disease%20(CVD)%20is%20one,%25%20CI%201.08%E2%80%932.02). https://
pmc.ncbi.nlm.nih.gov/articles/PMC6156407/ https://pmc.ncbi.nlm.nih.gov/articles/
PMC8564065/ https://www.ahajournals.org/doi/10.1161/circ.136.suppl_1.20249
106 https://www.researchgate.net/publication/5264727_Eating_Slowly_Led_to_
Decreases_in_Energy_Intake_within_Meals_in_Healthy_Women
107 https://www.sciencedirect.com/science/article/abs/pii/
S0950329324000971?via%3Dihub
108 https://pmc.ncbi.nlm.nih.gov/articles/PMC8840755/
109 https://pubmed.ncbi.nlm.nih.gov/35878732/
110 https://jn.nutrition.org/article/S0022-3166(23)00768-X/fulltext
111 https://pmc.ncbi.nlm.nih.gov/articles/PMC10453983/
112 https://pubmed.ncbi.nlm.nih.gov/18005489/
113 https://gut.bmj.com/content/68/1/83; https://journals.lww.com/md-journal/
fulltext/2018/10260/whole_grain_diet_reduces_systemic_inflammation__a.77.aspx
114 https://pubmed.ncbi.nlm.nih.gov/34255848/
115 https://pubmed.ncbi.nlm.nih.gov/30016529/

Live longer

116 https://ajcn.nutrition.org/article/S0002-9165(23)12516-0/fulltext
117 https://pmc.ncbi.nlm.nih.gov/articles/PMC4515860/
118 https://alz-journals.onlinelibrary.wiley.com/doi/10.1016/j.jalz.2017.01.024
119 https://pubmed.ncbi.nlm.nih.gov/30882235/
120 https://www.mayoclinic.org/healthy-lifestyle/nutrition-and-healthy-eating/in-depth/
fiber/art-20043983
121 https://pubmed.ncbi.nlm.nih.gov/37793780/
122 https://pmc.ncbi.nlm.nih.gov/articles/PMC1995688/
123 https://pubmed.ncbi.nlm.nih.gov/32514607/
124 https://pmc.ncbi.nlm.nih.gov/articles/PMC9156390/
125 https://www.cam.ac.uk/research/news/daily-11-minute-brisk-walk-enough-to-reduce-
risk-of-early-death
126 https://pmc.ncbi.nlm.nih.gov/articles/PMC4718793/
127 https://pmc.ncbi.nlm.nih.gov/articles/PMC7375895/#S13
128 https://pmc.ncbi.nlm.nih.gov/articles/PMC3804225/#S11
129 https://jamanetwork.com/journals/jamapediatrics/fullarticle/1655500

130 https://www.sciencedirect.com/science/article/pii/S0277953624009559?utm_
131 https://www.theatlantic.com/ideas/archive/2023/01/harvard-happiness-study-relationships/672753/
132 https://www.adultdevelopmentstudy.org/
133 https://haarc.center.uchicago.edu/superaging/
134 https://pubmed.ncbi.nlm.nih.gov/10776744
135 https://pubmed.ncbi.nlm.nih.gov/9200634/
136 https://pmc.ncbi.nlm.nih.gov/articles/PMC2910600
137 https://pubmed.ncbi.nlm.nih.gov/39158741/
138 https://www.amjmed.com/article/S0002-9343(14)00138-7/fulltext
139 https://pmc.ncbi.nlm.nih.gov/articles/PMC4617425/#sec5
140 https://journals.plos.org/plosone/article?id=10.1371/journal.pone.0000465
141 https://jamanetwork.com/journals/jamainternalmedicine/fullarticle/415534;
https://pubmed.ncbi.nlm.nih.gov/22529236/

Keep your heart healthy

142 http://www.asph.sc.edu/news/blair3.htm
143 https://pmc.ncbi.nlm.nih.gov/articles/PMC6803778/
144 https://pubmed.ncbi.nlm.nih.gov/22648725/
145 https://www.frontiersin.org/journals/nutrition/articles/10.3389/fnut.2022.1041203/full
146 https://www.sciencedirect.com/science/article/pii/S0002916523272470
147 https://www.researchgate.net/publication/365943504_Extra-Virgin_Olive_Oil_Enhances_the_Blood-Brain_Barrier_Function_in_Mild_Cognitive_Impairment_A_Randomized_Controlled_Trial
148 https://pmc.ncbi.nlm.nih.gov/articles/PMC4586551/
149 https://www.ncbi.nlm.nih.gov/pmc/articles/PMC5137931/
150 https://www.ncbi.nlm.nih.gov/pmc/articles/PMC6717875/
151 https://pubmed.ncbi.nlm.nih.gov/37174238/#:~:text=Participation%20in%20NW%20training%20also,physical%20activity%3B%20quality%20of%20health
152 https://pubmed.ncbi.nlm.nih.gov/34245777/
153 https://pubmed.ncbi.nlm.nih.gov/32243013/
154 https://www.sciencedirect.com/science/article/abs/pii/S0278691512008964
155 https://pmc.ncbi.nlm.nih.gov/articles/PMC3806204/#S27
https://www.sciencedirect.com/science/article/pii/S0022316623031978#:~:text=Recently%2C%20a%20longer%20follow%2Dup,with%20a%20strong%20genetic%20component
156 https://pubmed.ncbi.nlm.nih.gov/11340098/
157 http://news.bbc.co.uk/1/hi/health/7370759.stm
158 https://pmc.ncbi.nlm.nih.gov/articles/PMC4073186/
159 https://radar.brookes.ac.uk/radar/file/43c4340e-3269-450c-a76d-287e489e9b34/1/fulltext.pdf
160 https://pubmed.ncbi.nlm.nih.gov/21088453/
161 https://pubmed.ncbi.nlm.nih.gov/26458258/
162 https://www.sciencedirect.com/science/article/abs/pii/S0261561412001896
163 https://pubmed.ncbi.nlm.nih.gov/36250602/

Be stronger and fitter

164 https://pubmed.ncbi.nlm.nih.gov/27195456/
165 https://pubmed.ncbi.nlm.nih.gov/34391248/
166 https://linkinghub.elsevier.com/retrieve/pii/S1360859216301024
167 https://www.nhs.uk/live-well/exercise/pilates-and-yoga/pilates-for-beginners/
168 https://pure.hartpury.ac.uk/en/publications/effects-of-jumping-exercise-on-muscular-power-in-older-adults-a-m
169 http://pmc.ncbi.nlm.nih.gov/articles/PMC5722366/
170 https://pubmed.ncbi.nlm.nih.gov/24460005/#:~:text=Conclusion:%20After%2016%20weeks%20of,ethnicity;%20Target%20population:%20adults.
171 https://pubmed.ncbi.nlm.nih.gov/29578618/
172 https://core.ac.uk/download/pdf/197310365.pdf
173 https://pmc.ncbi.nlm.nih.gov/articles/PMC3755647/
174 https://pubmed.ncbi.nlm.nih.gov/30195124/#:~:text=Results:%20At%20baseline%2C%20the%20participants,a%20healthy%20lifestyle%20among%20adults.
175 https://pubmed.ncbi.nlm.nih.gov/17397428/
176 https://www.nature.com/articles/s41598-022-12526-5
177 https://www.acpjournals.org/doi/10.7326/M20-7014
178 https://www.bbc.co.uk/programmes/articles/4bW7dcH7WpKYVGprPSjJWWx/the-taste-of-tai-chi-challenge-makeyourmove
179 https://pubmed.ncbi.nlm.nih.gov/15776337/
180 https://pubmed.ncbi.nlm.nih.gov/8133744/
181 https://www.researchgate.net/publication/289267640_Backward_walking_A_possible_active_exercise_for_low_back_pain_reduction_and_enhanced_function_in_athletes
182 https://digitalcommons.wku.edu/ijes/vol4/iss3/4/
183 https://www.researchgate.net/publication/328149478_It_takes_me_back_The_mnemonic_time-travel_effect
184 https://journals.sagepub.com/doi/10.1111/j.1467-9280.2009.02342.x
185 https://www.unlv.edu/news/release/walking-backward-could-be-step-forward-elderly#:~:text=The%20project%20is%20conducted%20under,locomotion%20characteristics%20and%20reducing%20falls.
186 https://pubmed.ncbi.nlm.nih.gov/37555441/
187 https://pubmed.ncbi.nlm.nih.gov/35868813/
188 https://www.ucl.ac.uk/news/2023/jan/moderate-and-vigorous-physical-activity-most-critical-factor-boosting-mid-life-brain-power
189 https://pubmed.ncbi.nlm.nih.gov/35868813/
190 https://journals.lww.com/nsca-jscr/Fulltext/2013/03000/Integration_Core_Exercises_Elicit_Greater_Muscle.5.aspx
191 https://www.ijsr.net/getabstract.php?paperid=SR201011145832#:~:text=The%20Result%20showed%20significant%20effect,pain%2C%20improve%20quality%20of%20life
192 https://www.canterbury.ac.uk/news/2023/static-isometric-exercise-such-as-wall-sits-best-for-lowering-blood-pressure
193 https://pubmed.ncbi.nlm.nih.gov/34911677/

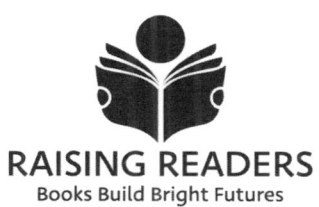

RAISING READERS
Books Build Bright Futures

Dear Reader,

We'd love your attention for one more page to tell you about the crisis in children's reading, and what we can all do.

Studies have shown that reading for fun is the **single biggest predictor of a child's future life chances** – more than family circumstance, parents' educational background or income. It improves academic results, mental health, wealth, communication skills, ambition and happiness.[1]

The number of children reading for fun is in rapid decline. Young people have a lot of competition for their time. In 2024, 1 in 10 children and young people in the UK aged 5 to 18 did not own a single book at home.[2]

Hachette works extensively with schools, libraries and literacy charities, but here are some ways we can all raise more readers:

- Reading to children for just 10 minutes a day makes a difference
- Don't give up if children aren't regular readers – there will be books for them!
- Visit bookshops and libraries to get recommendations
- Encourage them to listen to audiobooks
- Support school libraries
- Give books as gifts

There's a lot more information about how to encourage children to read on our website: **www.RaisingReaders.co.uk**

Thank you for reading.

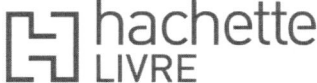

---

[1] OECD, '21st-Century Readers: Developing Literacy Skills in a Digital World', 2021, https://www.oecd.org/en/publications/21st-century-readers_a83d84cb-en.html

[2] National Literacy Trust, 'Book Ownership in 2024', November 2024. https://literacytrust.org.uk/research-services/research-reports/book-ownership-in-2024

First published in Great Britain in 2026
by Short Books, an imprint of
Octopus Publishing Group Ltd,
Carmelite House,
50 Victoria Embankment,
London EC4Y 0DZ
www.octopusbooks.co.uk

An Hachette UK Company
www.hachette.co.uk

The authorised representative in the
EEA is Hachette Ireland, 8 Castlecourt
Centre, Dublin 15, D15 XTP3, Ireland
(email: info@hbgi.ie)

Text copyright © BBC Studios Science Unit 2026
Illustrations copyright © Lindsey Spinks 2026

By arrangement with BBC Studios
Productions. The BBC and BBC Studios
logos are trademarks of the British
Broadcasting Corporation and are used
under licence. BBC and BBC Studios logos
© British Broadcasting Corporation.

Distributed in the US by Hachette Book
Group, 1290 Avenue of the Americas,
4th and 5th Floors, New York, NY 10104

Distributed in Canada by Canadian Manda
Group, 664 Annette St, Toronto, Ontario,
Canada M6S 2C8

All rights reserved. No part of this work
may be reproduced or utilised in any form
or by any means, electronic or mechanical,
including photocopying, recording or by
any information storage and retrieval system,
without the prior written permission of
the publisher.

Hardback ISBN: 9781804193938
Paperback ISBN: 9781804194034
eISBN: 9781804193945

A CIP catalogue record for this book
is available from the British Library.

Printed and bound in Great Britain.

10 9 8 7 6 5 4 3 2 1

Publisher: Jo Morrell
Commissioning Editor: Katie Forsythe
Editorial Consultant: Louise Atkinson
Senior Editor: Leanne Bryan
Copy Editor: Claudia Martin
Editorial Assistant: Sarah Ramnath Budhram
Creative Director: Mel Four
Designer: Jeremy Tilston
Illustrator: Lindsey Spinks
Production Controller: Sarah Parry

This FSC® label means that materials used for
the product have been responsibly sourced.

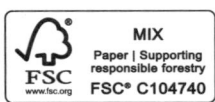

MIX
Paper | Supporting
responsible forestry
FSC® C104740

Note

The BBC does not endorse any specific product or service mentioned in this book.

Disclaimer

The chapter titles within this book are simplified summaries and not medical claims.

All reasonable care has been taken in the preparation of this book but the information
it contains is not intended to take the place of treatment by a qualified medical practitioner.

Before making any changes in your health regime, always consult a doctor, and if you are
struggling with your mental health, seek support from a qualified healthcare professional.
While all the therapies detailed in this book are completely safe if done correctly, you must
seek professional advice if you are in any doubt about any medical condition. Any application
of the ideas and information contained in this book is at the reader's sole discretion and risk.